Medical Assisting
Review

Medical Assisting Review

Marsha Perkins Hemby, BA, RN, CMA

Department Chairman, Medical Assisting
Pitt Community College
Greenville, North Carolina

Brady/Prentice Hall
Englewood Cliffs, New Jersey 07632

An American BookWorks Corporation Project
Contributing Editors: *Carolyn Lorandeau; Norma L. Forbrich*
Production Editor: *Cathy O'Connell*
Cover Design: *Marianne Frasco*
Prepress/Manufacturing Buyer: *Ilene Sanford*
Director of Manufacturing and Production: *Bruce Johnson*
Acquisitions Editor: *Barbara Krawiec*
Editorial Assistant: *Louise Fullam*
Printer/Binder: *Banta Company*

Thanks to Gene, my husband, who fixed the computer every time,
no matter the hour or the television program;
thanks to Jenny and Gene, Jr., for being patient with me, their Mom;
thanks to the Hills Point gang for keeping me sane;
and thanks, Fred, for getting me into this; It's been great!

Printed in the United States of America

10 9 8 7 6 5 4 3 2 1

ISBN   0835-4928-1

Prentice-Hall International (UK) Limited, *London*
Prentice-Hall of Australia Pty. Limited, *Sydney*
Prentice-Hall Canada Inc., *Toronto*
Prentice-Hall Hispanoamerica, S.A., *Mexico*
Prentice-Hall of India Private Limited, *New Delhi*
Prentice-Hall of Japan, Inc., *Tokyo*
Simon & Schuster Asia Pte. Ltd., *Singapore*
Editora Prentice-Hall do Brasil, Ltda., *Rio de Janeiro*

Contents

Preface   vii
How to use this Outline Book   ix
Introduction   xi

1   Medical terms and vocabulary   1

2   Anatomy and physiology   19

3   Professionalism   47

4   Patient communication   52

5   Medical law   56

6   Written communication   63

7   Office equipment   70

8   Medical records   76

9   Postal services   81

10 Appointment processes   85

11 Community services   90

12 Office management   93

13 Health insurance   101

14 Infection Control   107

15 Clinical equipment   116

16 Physician assisting   120

17 Laboratory procedures   135

18 Medication administration   148

19 Emergencies and first aid   167

Preface

The purpose of this book is review. It serves as a study guide for the Certification Examination for Medical Assistants. The book is an effort to review briefly, but as thoroughly as possible, critical areas of medical assisting using an outline format. This format is used to get as much information as possible in a concise manner. The "Content Outline of the American Association of Medical Assistants' Certification Examination" has been followed so that all areas of the exam will be addressed and reviewed. The book can be used as a review prior to the certification examination or as a source for teaching a review course prior to the examination.

The book is composed of an introductory chapter and nineteen chapters covering topics of the AAMA Content Outline. At the end of each chapter, there are questions for review and answers with explanations, which should assist in study and review for the examination.

How to Use This Outline Book

Imagine, if you will, the perfect set of class notes. You've gone to class every day, you've written down all the essential notes on the material that your instructor has taught, and you have even added some illustrations where appropriate. What could be better? This book is that complete set of notes!

Despite its streamlined appearance, it is an all-inclusive book. Every attempt has been made to include all the important points in the course, while eliminating much of the extraneous material that often is included. To make it easy for you to use, the book has been laid out in outline format. Like any outline, it is organized into various levels, and by glancing at the table of contents of this book, you will quickly learn how to use it.

All the books in this series have been developed by analyzing the existing textbooks in the field and the requirements of the specific accrediting organizations. From this analysis we have determined the key areas and topics to be included in the book. Thus this book is complete, which means that whether you are a student in California, Georgia, Maine, or Minnesota—any state in the country—regardless of what textbook you are using, this book will cover the material. This is important because you will want to use the book to help you review what you have learned, and of course you will want to be assured that the information you need is included here.

There is a step-by-step process involved in using any type of review book. First, you attend classroom lectures. Normally, there is a specific textbook designed for that class, and you are assigned chapters to read by your instructor. What happens, however, when you have attended class, read your textbook, but still find the information somewhat unclear? It's time to call on this outline book.

With this book's easy-to-use format, you can quickly identify the important ideas, concepts, and facts that are presented. Here is how the book is laid out:

A. This is the topic heading

    1. This is the first important point to be covered.

       a. Fact you should know

       b. A second fact you should know

    2. This is the second important point to be covered.

       a. Fact you should know

       b. A second fact you should know

Important terms are defined where necessary, and illustrations are included where they will help illuminate and clarify information.

Find the chapter in this book that corresponds to the topic in your textbook or to what you are covering in class. Read through the chapter quickly, skimming the material until you find the section that has given you difficulty. Now read through that part slowly. Underline or highlight words or phrases that you feel are important. It may be helpful to rewrite the information in your own words so it becomes even clearer to you. You might even want to make notes in the margins. Finally, compare this outline with your own class notes.

The concept of any review book is to make it easier to understand information you have learned elsewhere. The purpose of presenting this outline format is to make it even easier! These are your class notes —to read, to memorize, to annotate, and to help you understand everything you will need to do well in your course.

Introduction

Study Guides

Begin studying at least six weeks prior to the examination. Study the following guides, and if possible, try to take a review course.

1. *Content Outline and Candidate's Guide;* free copy of guide obtained from AAMA Certification Department, 20 North Wacker Drive, Suite 1575, Chicago, IL 60606-2903. Phone 1-800-228-2262; fax 1-312-899-1259.
2. *The Medical Assisting Examination Guide* by Lane, F.A. Davis Co., revised reprint, 1991.
3. *Medical Assistant Examination Review* by Dreizen and Audet, Medical Examination Publishing Co., 4th edition, 1989.
4. *The Medical Assistant, Administrative and Clinical* by Kinn, Woods, and Derge, W.B. Saunders, 7th edition, 1993.
5. *Comprehensive Medical Assisting* by Frew and Frew, F.A. Davis Co., 2nd edition, 1988.
6. *Fundamentals of Medical Assisting* by Zakus, C.V. Mosby, 2nd edition, 1990.
7. *Medical Assisting, Administrative and Clinical Competencies* by Kier and Wise, Delmar Publishers, 2nd edition, 1990.
8. *Medical Law, Ethics and Bioethics in the Medical Office* by Lewis and Tamparo, F.A. Davis Co., 3rd edition, 1993.
9. *Basic Laboratory Techniques* by Walters, Delmar Publishers, 2nd edition, 1990.
10. *Medical Terminology: A Short Course* by Chabner, W.B. Saunders, 1991.
11. *Clinical Procedures for Medical Assistants* by Bonewit, W.B. Saunders, 3rd edition, 1990.
12. *Saunders Manual of Medical Assisting Practice* by Lane, W.B. Saunders, 1993.
13. *The Medical Assisting Video Series*, Delmar Publishers, 1993.
14. *The Medical Assistant* by Cooper, Cooper, and Burrows, Mosby Lifeline, 6th edition, 1993.
15. *Fundamentals of Medical Assisting* by Zakus, Eggers, and Shea, C.V. Mosby, 2nd edition, 1990.

Test-Taking Tips

The CMA examination contains 300 questions: 100 each from the area of general, administrative, and clinical. The RMA examination contains 200 questions divided into equal parts of general, administrative, and clinical. The AAMT offers a voluntary certification by examination for medical transcriptionists. The CPS examination lasts two days and consists of six parts: Law, Economics and Managment, Accounting and Administration, Communications, Office Technology, and Business Behaviorial Science. Those passing become certified professional secretaries.

1. The first answer is usually the best answer unless the question has been misread.
2. Breakfast is a must! Test time is 9:00 AM to 1:00 PM for the CMA examination.
3. Entrance is allowed only with an admission ticket and photo ID for the CMA examination.
4. A number 2 pencil is to be supplied by the test-taker.
5. Mark items on the answer sheet totally; erase changes completely.
6. Less than 1 minute is allowed per question; you must pace yourself.
7. There is no penalty for guessing; mark all spaces.

Application Instructions

The RMA examination is given in March, June, and November at one location in each state; the CMA examination is given on the last Friday in January and June at 100 different locations; and the CPS examination is given in May and November.

DEADLINE FOR APPLICATIONS

CMA: March 1 for the June test, and October 1 for the January test
RMA: December 1 for the March test, March 1 for the June test, and August 1 for the November test

CMA (certified medical assistant):
1. Student or recent graduate of a CAHEA-accredited program or
2. Medical assisting instructor or
3. Experienced medical assistant or employee in health care field for one year full-time or two years part-time
Obtain applications from AAMA Certification Department, 20 North Wacker Drive, Suite 1575, Chicago, IL 60606-2903.

RMA (registered medical assistant):
1. High school graduate or equivalent
2. Graduate of a medical assisting program accredited by the Accrediting Bureau of Health Education Schools (ABHES) or a regional accrediting commission or
3. Formal medical training in the armed forces or
4. Medical assisting graduate of a program accredited by the Council

on Postsecondary Accreditation (COPA) and employed as a medical assistant for one year or

5. Employed as a medical assistant for five years

Obtain applications from American Medical Technologies, 710 Higgings Road, Park Ridge, IL 60068-5765. Phone: (708) 823-5169; fax: (708) 823-0458.

CPS information available from Professional Secretaries International, 301 East Armour Boulevard, Kansas City, MO 64111-1299.

AAMT information is available from the American Association for Medical Transcription, 3460 Oakdale Road, Suite D, P.O. Box 6187, Modesto, CA 95355.

Fees

CMA: $70 for a student/member; $145 for a nonmember (subject to change)
RMA: $59 (subject to change)
Both CMA and RMA require a certified check or money order.

1

Medical Terms and Vocabulary

CHAPTER OUTLINE

Word Structure
Definitions
Applications
Abbreviations
Body Planes, Divisions, and Directions

I. WORD STRUCTURE

Dividing a word into its root, prefix, suffix, and combining form, and understanding each part separately will ultimately help you discover the word's definition.

   A. *Root:* the main part of the word

   Example: hypo<u>gastr</u>ic: gastr- = root; gastr- means stomach

   B. *Prefix:* the first part of the word

   Example: <u>hypo</u>gastric: hypo- = prefix; hypo- means below
   hypogastric = below the stomach

   C. *Suffix:* the ending of the word

   Example: tonsill<u>itis</u>: -itis = suffix; -itis means inflammation of
   tonsillitis = inflammation of the tonsils

   D. *Combining form:* a word root plus a vowel

   Example: <u>cardio</u>logy: cardio- = combining form; cardio- means heart; -logy means study of
   cardiology = study of the heart

II. DEFINITIONS

   A. Prefixes

      1. Prefixes pertaining to position or placement
         a. ab- = away
         b. ad- = toward
         c. endo- = within
         d. epi- = above
         e. hyper- = above
         f. hypo- = below
         g. inter- = between
         h. retro- = behind, backward
         i. supra- = above

      2. Prefixes pertaining to amounts and time
         a. bi- = two
         b. brady- = slow
         c. hemi- = half
         d. poly- = many
         e. post- = after
         f. pre- = before
         g. quadri- = four
         h. tachy- = fast
         i. tri- = three

      3. Prefixes that are descriptive
         a. a- = not, negation
         b. anti- = against
         c. auto- = self
         d. dys- = difficult, painful, bad
         e. erythro- = red
         f. hemo- = blood

 g. histo- = tissue

 h. homeo- = same, alike

 i. hydro- = water

 j. litho- = stone

 k. mal- = bad

 l. melano- = black

 m. neo- = new

 n. pseudo- = false

4. Prefixes pertaining to parts of the body

 a. adeno- = gland

 b. arthro- = joint

 c. blepharo- = eyelid

 d. cardio- = heart

 e. cervico- = neck

 f. cranio- = skull

 g. cysto- = bladder

 h. cyto- = cell

 i. dermato- = skin

 j. hepato- = liver

 k. hystero- = uterus

 l. myelo- = marrow, spinal cord

B. Suffixes

1. -algia = pain; -dynia = pain

2. -blast = not developed; -genic = forming

3. -cele = swollen sac, protrusion; -cyte = cell; -oma = tumor, growth; -lith = stone

4. -centesis = removal of fluid by puncturing

5. -cide = causing death

6. -ectomy = cutting out; -tomy = cutting; -plasty = surgical repair; -rrhaphy = suturing

7. -emesis = vomiting

8. -emia = blood condition

9. -gram = written record

10. -itis = inflammation of; -osis = diseased; -pathy = diseased; -plegia = paralysis

11. -lysis = destruction of, breaking apart; -desis = fixing together

12. -malacia = softening of; -sclerosis = hardening of

13. -megaly = enlarged

14. -mimetic = imitation

15. -opia = vision; -scopy = viewing

16. -penia = deficiency

17. -phagia = swallowing; -pnea = breathing

18. -rhea = discharge; -rhagia = bursting forth (also -rrhea, -rrhagia)

C. Combining forms
  1. Combining forms pertaining to parts of the body
     a. angio- = vessel
     b. cephalo- = head
     c. costo- = rib
     d. glosso- = tongue
     e. kerato- = cornea, horny layer
     f. laparo- = abdomen
     g. myo- = muscle
     h. neuro- = nerve
     i. oculo- = eyes
     j. osteo- = bone
     k. oto- = ear
     l. phlebo- = vein
     m. pyelo- = pelvis
     n. rhino- = nose
     o. stomato- = mouth
     p. veno- = vein
  2. Combining forms pertaining to organs
     a. cholecysto- = gallbladder
     b. encephalo- = brain
     c. entero- = intestines
     d. gastro- = stomach
     e. nephr- = kidney
     f. pneum- = air in the lungs
     g. procto- = rectum
     h. pulmo- = lungs
  3. Descriptive combining forms
     a. audio- = hearing
     b. chromo- = color
     c. cyano- = blue
     d. diplo- = double
     e. iatro- = related to medicine or physician
     f. leuko- = white
     g. lipo- = fat
     h. macro- = large
     i. micro- = small
     j. morpho- = shape
     k. nocto- = night
     l. oligo- = scant
     m. onco- = tumor
     n. ortho- = straight
     o. patho- = disease
     p. thrombo- = clot

III. APPLICATIONS

A. Prefixes pertaining to position or placement
1. ab- = away
   a. abrade = scrape away
   b. ablation = taking away of a part
2. ad- = toward
   a. adrenal = toward the kidney
   b. adduct = move a part toward the body
3. endo- = within
   a. endocarditis = inflammation within the inner lining of the heart
   b. endoscope = instrument for viewing within an organ or cavity
4. epi- = above
   a. epigastric = above the stomach
   b. epinephrine = hormone secreted by the adrenal glands above the kidney
5. hyper- = above, excessive
   a. hyperthermia = above-normal temperature
   b. hypertension = above-normal pressure
6. hypo- = below
   a. hypogastric = below the stomach
   b. hypodermic = needle injected below the skin
7. inter- = between
   a. intercostal = between the ribs
   b. interarticular = between the joints
8. retro- = behind, backward
   a. retrograde = moving or flowing backward
   b. retrolingual = behind the tongue
9. supra- = above
   a. supraorbital = above the eye's orbit
   b. suprapubic = above the pubic arch

B. Prefixes pertaining to amounts and time
1. bi- = two
   a. biceps = muscle with two heads
   b. bicuspid = having two cusps or flaps, as in the bicuspid valve of the heart
2. brady- = slow
   a. bradycardia = slow rhythm of the heart
   b. bradypnea = slow breathing
3. hemi- = half
   a. hemiplegia = paralysis of one-half of the body
   b. hemifacial = pertaining to one-half of the face
4. poly- = many
   a. polyarthritis = many inflamed joints
   b. polydactylism = extra fingers and toes

5. post- = after
   a. postoperative = after an operation
   b. postpartum = after the birth of a baby
6. pre- = before
   a. prenatal = before the birth of a baby
   b. premenstrual = before menstruation
7. quadri- = four
   a. quadriplegic = four limbs paralyzed
   b. quadriceps = muscle with four heads
8. tachy- = fast
   a. tachycardia = fast rhythm of the heart
   b. tachypnea = fast breathing
9. tri- = three
   a. triceps = muscle with three heads but one insertion
   b. tricuspid = valve between the right atrium and ventricle that has three cusps

C. Prefixes that are descriptive
1. a- = not, negation
   a. afebrile = no fever
   b. asepsis = not contaminated
2. anti- = against
   a. antibacterial = against bacteria
   b. anticoagulant = against the forming of clots
3. auto- = self
   a. autonomic = self-controlling, as in autonomic nervous system
   b. autograft = graft of one's self
4. dys- = difficulty, painful, bad
   a. dyspnea = difficulty in breathing
   b. dyspepsia = difficulty in digesting
5. erythro- = red
   a. erythrocyte = red blood cell
   b. erythropoiesis = red blood cell formation
6. hemo- = blood
   a. hemoptysis = spitting up of blood
   b. hemolysis = destruction of blood cells
7. histo- = tissue
   a. histology = study of tissues
   b. histokinesis = movement of tissue in the body
8. homeo- = same, like
   a. homeostasis = staying the same
   b. homeoosteoplasty = grafting of bone similar to bone upon which it is grafted
9. hydro- = water
   a. hydrotherapy = treatment using water
   b. hydrocephalus = increased fluid in the brain

10. litho- = stone
    a. lithotripsy = crushing of stones ✗
    b. lithuresis = passing of stones while urinating
11. mal- = bad
    a. malpractice = bad practice
    b. malnutrition = bad nutrition
12. melano- = black
    a. melanopathy = dark pigmentation of the skin ✗
    b. melanoglossia = black tongue
13. neo- = new
    a. neonatal = newborn
    b. neoplasm = new growing thing
14. pseudo- = false
    a. pseudotumor = symptoms like a tumor, but not a tumor
    b. pseudoplegia = paralysis of hysterical origin ✓

D. Prefixes pertaining to parts of the body
    1. adeno- = gland
        a. adenoma = tumor of a gland
        b. adenitis = inflammation of a gland
    2. arthro- = joint
        a. arthroplasty = plastic surgery of a joint
        b. arthrodesis = surgical fixation or fusion of a joint
    3. blepharo- = eyelid
        a. blepharospasm = twitching of the eyelid
        b. blepharoptosis = drooping of the eyelid ✓
    4. cardio- = heart
        a. cardiologist = one who studies and specializes in the heart
        b. cardiogram = written record of the heart's activity
    5. cervico- = neck
        a. cervicodynia = neck pain
        b. cervicofacial = pertaining to the face and neck
    6. cranio- = skull
        a. craniotomy = incision into the skull
        b. craniocele = protrusion of part of the brain into the skull
    7. cysto- = bladder
        a. cystoscopy = viewing and examining the bladder
        b. cystitis = inflammation of the bladder
    8. cyto- = cell
        a. cytologist = one who studies cells
        b. cytogeny = formation of a cell
    9. dermato- = skin
        a. dermatitis = inflammation of the skin
        b. dermatology = study of the skin

10. hepato- = liver
    a. hepatomegaly = enlarged liver
    b. hepatoma = liver tumor
11. hystero- = uterus
    a. hysterectomy = cutting out of the uterus
    b. hysterorrhexis = uterine rupture
12. myelo- = marrow, spinal cord
    a. myeloma = tumor beginning in the blood-forming part of the marrow
    b. myelopathy = disease of the spinal cord

E. Suffixes
    1. -algia=pain; -dynia = pain
        a. neuralgia = pain along the course of a nerve
        b. myalgia = muscle tenderness and pain
        c. cephalodynia = pain in the head
        d. gastrodynia = stomach pain
    2. -blast=not developed; -genic = forming
        a. erythroblast = immature red blood cell
        b. neuroblast = embryonic cell
        c. neurogenesis = forming of nerves
        d. cardiogenic = originating in the heart
    3. -cele = swollen sac or protrusion; -cyte = cell; -oma = tumor
        a. cystocele = protrusion of the bladder into the vaginal wall
        b. rectocele = protrusion of the rectal wall into the vaginal wall
        c. erythrocyte = red blood cell
        d. leukocyte = white blood cell
        e. carcinoma = malignant tumor arising from epithelial tissue
        f. sarcoma = tumor arising from connective tissue
    4. -centesis = removal of fluid by puncturing
        a. paracentesis = puncture of a cavity with removal of fluid
        b. arthrocentesis = removal of fluid from a joint by needle puncture
    5. cide = causing death
        a. sporicide = spore-destroying agent
        b. bacteriocide = bacteria-destroying agent
    6. -ectomy = cutting out, excision of; -tomy = cutting; -rrhaphy = suturing; -plasty = surgical repair; -pexy = fixation of
        a. appendectomy = cutting out of appendix
        b. hysterectomy = cutting out of uterus
        c. cystotomy = incision of bladder
        d. myotomy = dissection of muscles
        e. hysterotrachelorrhaphy = paring the edges and suturing of the lacerated cervix
        f. laparorrhaphy = suturing of a wound inside the abdominal wall

    g. pyloroplasty = surgery of the portion of the stomach that connects to the duodenum

    h. hernioplasty = surgical repair of a hernia

    i. cystopexy = surgical fixation of the bladder to the wall of abdomen

    j. nephropexy = surgical fixation of a kidney

7. -emesis = vomiting

    a. hematemesis = vomiting of blood

    b. pyemesis = vomiting of pus

8. -emia = blood condition

    a. anemia = blood condition with reduced red blood cells, packed cells, and hemoglobin

    b. pyemia = condition with pus-forming organisms in the blood

9. -gram = written record

    a. cardiogram = written record of the heart's electrical activity

    b. electroencephalogram = written record of the brain's waves

10. -itis = inflammation of; -osis = diseased; -pathy = diseased; -plegia = paralysis

    a. arthritis = inflammation of the joints

    b. blepharitis = inflammation of the eyelids

    c. stomatosis = any diseased condition of the mouth

    d. keratosis = diseased cornea

    e. myopathy = disease of a muscle

    f. neuropathy = disease of the nerves

    g. hemiplegia = paralysis on one side

    h. quadriplegia = paralysis of all four limbs and the trunk

11. -lysis = destruction of, breaking apart; -desis = fixing together; -tripsy = crushing of

    a. hemolysis = destruction of blood cells

    b. carcinolysis = destruction of cancer cells

    c. arthrodesis = surgical immobilization of a joint

    d. lithotripsy = crushing of stones (calculili)

    e. neurotripsy = surgical crushing of a nerve

12. -malacia = softening; -sclerosis=hardening of

    a. osteomalacia = softening of the bones

    b. neuromalacia = softening of neural tissue

    c. arteriosclerosis = hardening of the arteries

    d. otosclerosis = hardening of the bone conductors of sound in the ear

13. -megaly = enlarged

    a. splenomegaly = enlarged spleen

    b. cardiomegaly = enlarged heart

14. -mimetic = imitation
   a. sympathomimetic = imitating the sympathetic nervous system
15. -opia = vision; -scopy = viewing
   a. myopia = best vision is very close vision
   b. diplopia = double vision
   c. arthroscopy = viewing of a joint
   d. laparoscopy = viewing inside the abdominal cavity
16. -penia = deficiency
   a. thrombocytopenia = deficiency of platelets
   b. erythrocytopenia = deficiency of red blood cells
17. -phagia = swallowing; -pnea = breathing
   a. dysphagia = difficulty in swallowing
   b. dyspnea = difficulty in breathing
   c. apnea = a period of no breathing
18 -rhea = discharge; -rhagia = bursting forth (also -rrhea, -rrhagia)
   a. diarrhea = discharge or excessive flow from the bowels
   b. gastrorrhea = excessive discharge of the gastric juices
   c. hemorrhagia = bursting forth of blood
   d. metrorrhagia = bleeding from the uterus (not during normal menses)

F. Combining forms pertaining to parts of the body
   1. angio- = vessel
      a. angioplasty = plastic surgery of a blood vessel
      b. angiography = radiography of blood vessels
   2. cephalo- = head
      a. cephalgia = headache
      b. cephalomotor = pertaining to movement of the head
   3. costo- = rib
      a. intercostal = between the ribs
      b. costectomy = resection of a rib
   4. glosso- = tongue
      a. glossopharyngeal = relating to the tongue and pharynx
      b. glossopathy = disease of the tongue
   5. kerato- = cornea, horny layer
      a. keratotomy = incision of the cornea
      b. keratoplasty = plastic surgery of the cornea
   6. laparo- = abdomen
      a. laparoscopy = viewing and examining the abdominal cavity
      b. laparorrhaphy = suturing of wounds within the abdominal wall
   7. myo- = muscle
      a. myoplasty = plastic surgery of muscle tissue
      b. myoma = tumor of muscle tissue

8. neuro- = nerve
    a. neuropathy = diseased nerve
    b. neurotripsy = crushing of a nerve
9. oculo- = eyes
    a. ocular = pertaining to the eyes
    b. oculomotor = relating to eye movements
10. osteo- = bone
    a. osteomalacia = softening of a bone
    b. osteotome = cutting instrument for the bone
11. oto- = ear
    a. otoscope = instrument for viewing the ears
    b. otosclerosis = hardening of the conduction parts of the ear
12. phlebo- = vein
    a. phlebogram = tracing of venous pulse
    b. phlebitis = inflammation of a vein
13. pyelo- = pelvis
    a. pyelopathy = any disease of the kidney's pelvis
    b. pyelonephritis = inflammation of the kidney and the kidney's pelvis
14. rhino- = nose
    a. rhinoplasty = plastic surgery of the nose
    b. rhinitis = inflammation of the nose
15. stomato- = mouth
    a. stomatitis = inflammation of the mouth
    b. stomatosis = any disease of the mouth
16. veno- = vein
    a. intravenous = within the vein
    b. venation = distribution of veins in a structure

G. Combining forms pertaining to the organs
    1. cholecysto- = gallbladder
        a. cholecystolithiasis = gallstones in the gallbladder
        b. cholecystectomy = cutting out the gallbladder
    2. encephalo- = brain
        a. encephalitis = inflammation of the brain
        b. encephalomalacia = softening of the brain
    3. entero- = intestines
        a. enterocentesis = puncture of the intestines to remove fluid
        b. enteritis = inflammation of the intestines
    4. gastro- = stomach
        a. gastroenterology = study of the stomach and intestines
        b. gastrocele = hernia or protrusion of the stomach
    5. nephro- = kidney
        a. nephrectomy = cutting out the kidney
        b. nephrolith = kidney stone

6. pneum- = pertaining to respiration and air in the lungs
   a. pneumothorax = air in the pleural cavity of a lung
   b. pneumogram = record of respirations and air movement
7. procto = rectum
   a. proctoscopy = viewing of the rectum
   b. proctology = the study of the rectum
8. pulmo = lung
   a. cardiopulmonary = pertaining to the heart and lungs
   b. pulmonitis = inflammation of the lungs

H. Combining forms that are descriptive
1. audio- = hearing
   a. audiometer = machine that tests hearing
   b. audiologist = one who studies hearing
2. chromo- = color
   a. chromoturia = abnormal coloring of urine
   b. chromotherapy = using colored light as a disease treatment
3. cyano- = blue
   a. cyanosis = blue discoloration
   b. cyanopia = vision when all appears blue
4. diplo- = double
   a. diplopia = double vision
   b. diplococci = round bacteria in pairs
5. iatro- = medicine or physician related
   a. iatrogeny = condition induced by a physician
   b. iatrotechniques = art of medicine and surgery
6. leuko- = white
   a. leukocyte = white blood cell
   b. leukoplakia = white patches on the tongue and inside the cheek
7. lipo- = fat
   a. liposuction = suctioning out of fat
   b. lipoblast = immature fat cell
8. macro- = large
   a. macromastia = abnormally large breastss
   b. macrotia = abnormally large ears
9. micro- = small
   a. microcephalus = abnormally small head
   b. microdont = having very small teeth
10. morpho- = shape
    a. morphology = study of shapes
    b. morphometry = measurement of forms
11. nocto- = night
    a. nocturia = frequent urinating at night
    b. noctiphobia = fear of the night and darkness

12. oligo- = scant, slight amount
    a. oliguria = scant amount of urine
    b. oligodipsia = abnormal decrease in the desire for fluids
13. onco- = tumor
    a. oncology = study of tumors
    b. oncogenesis = tumor formation
14. ortho- = straight, normal, correct
    a. orthopnea = cannot breathe well unless standing or sitting straight
    b. orthopedics = pertaining to the correction of deformities
15. patho- = disease
    a. pathology = study of disease
    b. pathogen = substance that is capable of producing disease
16. thrombo- = clot
    a. thrombocyte = clot-producing cell; platelet
    b. thrombolysis = destruction of a clot

IV. ABBREVIATIONS

A. Abbreviations: medication administration
   1. a.c. = before meals
   2. ad lib = as needed
   3. A.D. = right ear
   4. A.S. = left ear
   5. A.U. = both ears, each ear
   6. b.i.d. = twice a day
   7. gtt. = drop
   8. h. = hour
   9. h.s. = bedtime, hour of sleep
   10. IM = intramuscular
   11. N.P.O. = nothing by mouth
   12. O.D. = right eye
   13. O.S. = left eye
   14. O.U. = both eyes, each eye
   15. p.c. = after meals
   16. P.O. = by mouth
   17. q.d. = every day
   18. q.h. = every hour
   19. q.i.d. = four times a day
   20. q.o.d. = every other day
   21. SC = subcutaneous
   22. stat. = immediately
   23. t.i.d. = three times a day

B. Abbreviations: medical diagnoses
   1. ASCVD = arteriosclerotic cardiovascular disease
   2. CA = cancer
   3. CHF = congestive heart failure
   4. COPD = chronic obstructive pulmonary disease
   5. CVA = cerebrovascular accident
   6. DM = diabetes mellitus; IDDM = insulin-dependent diabetes mellitus; NIDDM = non-insulin-dependent diabetes mellitus
   7. MI = myocardial infarction
   8. MS = multiple sclerosis
   9. R.A. = rheumatoid arthritis
   10. TB = tuberculosis
   11. TIA = transient ischemic attack
   12. URI = upper respiratory infection
   13. UTI = urinary tract infection
C. Miscellaneous abbreviations
   1. A and W = alive and well
   2. BM = bowel movement
   3. BP = blood pressure
   4. Bx = biopsy
   5. D and C = dilation and curettage
   6. DOA = dead on arrival
   7. DOB = date of birth
   8. Dx = diagnosis
   9. ENT = ear, nose, throat
   10. FU = follow-up
   11. Fx = fracture
   12. K = potassium
   13. N/V = nausea and vomiting
   14. ROS = review of systems
   15. SOB = shortness of breath
   16. UA = urinalysis
   17. VA = visual acuity

V. BODY PLANES, DIVISIONS, AND DIRECTIONS
   A. _Body planes_
      1. _Frontal (coronal):_ divides the body into front and back (anterior and posterior); anterior = ventral, posterior = dorsal
      2. _Transverse:_ divides the body (at the waist) into upper and lower (superior and inferior)
      3. _Midsagittal:_ divides the body into right and left sides
   B. _Divisions:_ the abdomen is divided into four divisions with the umbilicus (navel) as the center.
      1. _Right upper quadrant (RUQ):_ right upper area of the abdomen; contains parts of the liver, gallbladder, and intestines.

2. *Left upper quadrant (LUQ):* left upper area of the abdomen; contains parts of the liver, stomach, pancreas, spleen, and intestines.
3. *Right lower quadrant (RLQ):* right lower area of the abdomen; contains parts of the intestines, appendix, right ureter, ovary, and fallopian tube.
4. *Left lower quadrant (LLQ):* left lower abdominal area; contains parts of the intestines, left ureter, ovary, and fallopian tube.

C. *Regions:* the abdomen is divided like a tic-tac-toe board with the umbilicus in the center.
   1. *Top two side squares:* right and left hypochondriac regions
   2. *Bottom two side squares:* right and left inguinal (iliac) regions
   3. *Top middle square:* epigastric region
   4. *Middle two side squares:* right and left lateral regions
   5. *Center square:* umbilical region
   6. *Lower middle square:* hypogastric region

D. Directions
   1. *Distal:* at the end of a structure; the insertion of a muscle is at the distal end
   2. *Proximal:* at the beginning of a structure; at the origin of a muscle
   3. *Lateral:* side
   4. *Medial:* middle
   5. *Anterior (ventral):* front, in front of
   6. *Posterior (dorsal):* back, in back of
   7. *Inferior (caudal):* lower, below
   8. *Superior (cephalic):* at the head, above

E. *Anatomical position:* the body is erect and standing with hands at sides, and palms forward.

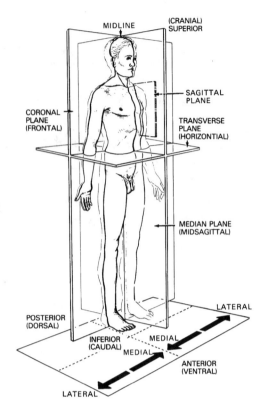

Figure 1-1 Anatomical direction and planes.

Match the key word with the proper combining form.

1. Joint
   a. thrombo-
   b. clavico-
   c. costo-
   d. arthro- *Join*
   e. scapulo-

2. Nose
   a. oto-
   b. rhino- *Nose*
   c. laryngo-
   d. cheilo-
   e. blepharo-

3. Bladder, sac
   a. cyto-
   b. colo-
   c. onco-
   d. uretero-
   e. cysto- *bladder*

4. Mouth
   a. stomato- *mouth*
   b. salpingo-
   c. cervico-
   d. cholecysto-
   e. dacryo-

5. Vessel
   a. veno-
   b. angio- *vessel*
   c. myo-
   d. tricho-
   e. viscero-

6. Kidney, pelvis
   a. procto-
   b. metro-
   c. entero-
   d. pyelo- *kidney*
   e. pyo-

7. Stomach
   a. stomato-
   b. lipo-
   c. gastro- *stomach*
   d. hystero-
   e. myelo-

8. Red
   a. leuko-
   b. erythro- *red*
   c. cyano-
   d. melano-
   e. hemo-

9. Liver
   a. masto-
   b. sacro-
   c. nephro-
   d. hepato- *Liver*
   e. pneumo-

10. Toward
    a. a-
    b. ab-
    c. ad- *toward*
    d. pro-
    e. di-

11. Two
    a. quadri-
    b. tri-
    c. mono-
    d. bi- *two*
    e. poly-

12. Within
    a. trans-
    b. retro-
    c. intra- *within*
    d. inter-
    e. epi-

13. Difficult
    a. dys- *difficult*
    b. mal-
    c. tachy-
    d. brady-
    e. hyper-

14. Pain
    a. -dynia
    b. -pexy
    c. -spasm
    d. -rrhea
    e. -pathy

15. Visual examination
    a. -ptosis
    b. oculo-
    c. -scopy
    d. -tomy
    e. -centesis

16. Fixation or binding of
    a. -desis
    b. -rrhaphy
    c. -tripsy
    d. -lysis
    e. iatro-

17. Softening of
    a. -sclerosis
    b. -phagia
    c. -megaly
    d. -malacia
    e. -penia

18. Scant, slight
    a. kerato-
    b. histo-
    c. neo-
    d. -itis
    e. oligo-

Answers

1. d arthro- = joint
   thrombo- = clot; clavico- = collar bone;
   costo- = rib; scapulo- = shoulder blade

2. b rhino- = nose
   oto- = ear; laryngo- = larynx; cheilo- = lip;
   blepharo- = eyelid

3. e cysto- = bladder
   cyto- = cell; colo- = colon; onco- = tumor;
   uretero- = ureter

4. a stomato- = mouth
   salpingo- = tube; cervico- = neck or
   cervix; cholecysto- = gallbladder, dacryo-
   = tears

5. b angio- = vessel
   veno- = vein; myo- = muscle; tricho- = hair;
   viscero- = relating to organs of the body

6. d pyelo- = kidney, pelvis
   procto- = rectum; metro- = uterus;
   entero- = intestines; pyo- = pus

7. c gastro- = stomach
   stomato- = mouth; lipo- = fat; hystero-
   = uterus; myelo = marrow, spinal cord

8. b erythro- = red
   leuko- = white; cyano- = blue; melano-
   = black; hemo- = blood

9. d hepato- = liver
   masto- = breast; sacro- = sacrum; nephro-
   = kidney; pneumo = air, respirations, lungs

10. c ad- = toward
    a- = not, negation; ab- = away from; pro-
    = before; di- = twice, double

11. d bi- = two
    quadri- = four; tri- = three; mono- = one;
    poly- = many

12. c intra- = within
    trans- = across; retro- = backward,
    behind; inter- = between; epi- = upon, over

13. a dys- = difficult
    mal- = bad; tachy- = fast; brady- = slow;
    hyper- = above, excessive

14. a -dynia = pain
    -pexy = fixation; -spasm = involuntary
    contraction; -rrhea = discharge; -pathy
    = disease

15. c -scopy = visual examination
    -ptosis = drooping; oculo- = eyes; -tomy
    = process of cutting; -centesis = removing
    fluid by puncture

16. a -desis = fixation or binding of
    -rhaphy = suturing; -tripsy = crushing;
    -lysis = destruction of or breaking
    away; iatro- = physician-related

17. d -malacia = softening of
    -sclerosis = hardening of; -phagia = swal-
    lowing; -megaly = enlarged; -penia = defi-
    ciency

18. e oligo- = scant, slight
    kerato- = cornea or horny layer;
    histo- = tissue; neo- = new; -itis = inflam-
    mation of

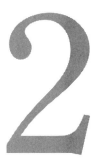

Anatomy and Physiology

Systems are made up of organs; organs are made up of tissue; and tissues are made up of cells.

CHAPTER OUTLINE

Integumentary System
Skeletal System
Muscular System
Digestive System
Cardiovascular System/Lymphatic System
Respiratory System
Nervous System/Special Senses
Urinary System
Reproductive System
Endocrine System

I. INTEGUMENTARY SYSTEM

For diseases of the integumentary system, one would visit the dermatologist.

  A. Anatomy of the skin

      1. *Epidermis:* outermost layer of the skin

      2. *Dermis:* middle layer of the skin, contains:

         a. *Sweat glands:* same as sudoriferous glands: secrete sweat or sudor

         b. *Sebaceous glands:* secrete sebum, an oily, fatty substance

         c. *Nerves and nerve endings*

         d. *Blood vessels*

      3. *Subcutaneous:* innermost layer, the tissue below the dermis

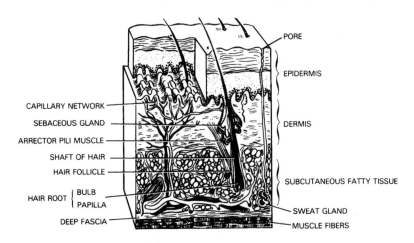

Figure 2-1 The integumentary system.

  B. Physiology of the skin

      1. *Epidermis*

         a. Barrier from the outside: therefore is protective

         b. Receptor for touch

         c. Preventer of water loss

      2. *Dermis*

         a. Temperature regulator: heat escapes through blood vessel expansion and release of sweat through the pores to cool body surfaces

         b. *Sebum:* keeps skin oiled and elastic and prevents dry hair and scalp

      3. *Subcutaneous*

         a. Provider for body fuel

         b. Retainer of heat

         c. Cushion for inner tissues

C. Diseases and conditions
   1. *Erythema:* reddened skin
   2. *Cyanosis:* blueness of the skin
   3. *Jaundice:* yellowed skin
   4. *Vitiligo:* white patches of the skin
   5. *Acne vulgaris:* inflamed follicles of the sebaceous glands
   6. *Dermatitis/eczema:* any acute or chronic skin inflammation
   7. *Impetigo:* contagious skin infection usually caused by streptococcus or staphylococcus
   8. *Psoriasis:* chronic red raised areas of the skin that are scaly and itchy; may progress into silver-yellow scales
   9. *Ringworm:* fungus affecting the scalp, feet, groin, or the body in general
   10. *Scabies:* infection caused by a mite that burrows under the skin, causing itching
   11. *Urticaria:* hives or raised wheals caused by an allergic reaction or stress
D. Diagnostics and procedures
   1. *Wood's light:* fluorescent purple light used to diagnose certain skin conditions
   2. *Diascope:* flat glass plate held against the skin to examine superficial skin lesions
   3. *Surgical excision and biopsy:* cutting out a lesion, mole, or skin cancer, and examining it under the microscope to identify cancerous cells
   4. *Sweat chloride test:* salt content of sweat: diagnostic for cystic fibrosis

II. SKELETAL SYSTEM

For diseases of the skeletal system, one would visit the orthopedist; for joints, the rheumatologist.
A. Bone anatomy (approximately 206 bones)
   1. *Skull:* head bone (cranium); joints of the cranium are called sutures
      a. *Frontal bone:* forehead and eye sockets
      b. *Temporal bones:* both sides around the ear and lower jaw
      c. *Parietal bones:* each side above the temporal bone
      d. *Occipital bone:* back of the head and base of the skull
   2. *Scapula:* upper back bone (shoulder blade) (not to be confused with scalpel, a surgical instrument used for cutting)
   3. *Clavicle:* anterior shoulder bone (collar bone)
   4. *Humerus:* upper arm bone
   5. *Radius:* lower arm bone on the thumb side
   6. *Ulna:* lower arm bone on the little finger side
   7. *Femur:* upper e ribone; longest and strongest of the bones
   8. *Tibia:* lower e r; largest of the lower eeg bones (shin bone)

9. *Fibula:* smallest of the lower leg bones; lower lateral bone of the leg
10. *Tarsals:* ankle bones (calcaneus is the heel bone)
11. *Metatarsals:* bones in the foot

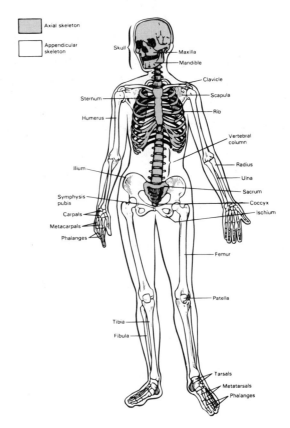

Axial skeleton
Appendicular skeleton

Skull
Maxilla
Mandible
Clavicle
Sternum
Scapula
Rib
Humerus
Vertebral column
Radius
Ilium
Ulna
Sacrum
Coccyx
Symphysis pubis
Ischium
Carpals
Metacarpals
Phalanges
Femur
Patella
Tibia
Fibula
Tarsals
Metatarsals
Phalanges

Figure 2-2 The skeletal system.

12. *Carpals:* wrist bones
13. *Metacarpals:* hand bones
14. *Phalanges:* finger and toe bones
15. *Patella:* knee bone
16. *Sternum:* upper middle of chest; ribs connect to the sternum, and CPR chest compression is done here
    a. *Xiphoid process:* lowest portion of the sternum
17. *Vertebrae*
    a. *Cervical:* seven bones curve inward; atlas is the top bone
    b. *Thoracic:* twelve bones curve outward
    c. *Lumbar:* five bones curve inward
    d. *Sacral:* five fused bones curve outward
    e. *Coccygeal:* four fused bones
18. *Smallest bones in body:* malleus, incus, and stapes (bones in ear)
19. *Greater trochanter:* "knob" or muscle attachment process at the top of the femur
20. *Pelvis:* basin-shaped structure formed by the ilium, ischium, pubis, sacrum, coccyx, and ligaments

B. Physiology
   1. Support for the body
   2. Protection of internal organs
   3. Movement of the body and joints
   4. Attachment for muscles
   5. Formation of red blood cells in the bone marrow
   6. Storage for calcium
C. Diseases and conditions
   1. *Fracture:* breaking of a bone
      a. *Greenstick:* incomplete break, like a green stick
      b. *Simple:* broken bone that does not break through the skin
      c. *Compound:* broken bone that breaks through the skin
      d. *Impacted:* broken ends of the bone penetrate into each other
      e. *Spiral:* twisted break
      f. *Comminuted:* more than one piece of the bone is broken
   2. *Arthritis:* inflammation of joints
   3. *Gout:* painful condition usually affecting the big toe; caused by uric acid buildup
   4. *Curvature of the spine:* lordosis (inward/swayback), kyphosis (outward/hunchback), and scoliosis (lateral/sideward)
   5. *Sprain:* tearing of ligaments
   6. *Carpal tunnel syndrome:* pressure on the median nerve in the carpal tunnel of the wrist
   7. *Rickets:* lack of vitamin D, causing softening of the bones
   8. *Osteoporosis:* reduction of bone mass, interfering with support
   9. *Osteomalacia:* softening of bone, causing deformities, pain, and weakness
D. Diagnostics and procedures
   1. *X-ray:* picture of bones to check breaks, density, and so on
   2. *Laminectomy and spinal fusion:* removing part of a vertebrae in order to remove a protrusion of the disk and fusing the area to stabilize it
   3. *Arthroscopy:* viewing of a joint; can also provide surgical access
   4. *Arthrocentesis:* puncture, usually for removal of fluid in a joint for analysis, or for relief of pain caused by pressure
   5. *Traction and reduction:* pulling on opposite ends of a bone to realign the bone

III. MUSCULAR SYSTEM

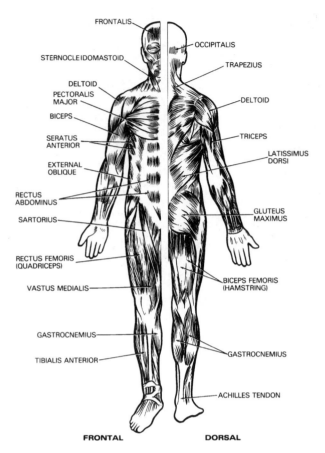

Figure 2-3 The muscular system.

For conditions of the muscular system, one would see an orthopedist; for therapy, a physical therapist.

A. Muscle anatomy (more than 600 muscles)

1. *Skeletal muscles:* voluntary movement; controlled by the cerebral cortex

   a. *Biceps:* upper arm bender or flexor

   b. *Triceps:* upper arm straightener or extensor

   c. *Pectoralis major:* chest muscle

   d. *Deltoid:* upper shoulder and arm muscle; site for injections

   e. *Gluteus medius:* buttocks muscle; upper outer quadrant used for injections at the dorsogluteal or ventrogluteal site

   f. *Vastus lateralis:* upper outer thigh; injection site, especially for infants

2. *Smooth muscles:* involuntary control

3. *Cardiac muscles:* automatic and rhythmic

4. *Ligaments:* attach bone to bone

5. *Tendons:* attach muscle to bone

   a. *Achilles tendon:* ankle; strongest tendon and site of ankle-jerk reflex

B. _Muscle physiology:_ contraction and relaxation enabling movement

    1. _Abduction:_ movement away from the body

    2. _Adduction:_ movement toward the body

C. Diseases and conditions

    1. _Tendonitis:_ inflammation of the tendons

    2. _Epicondylitis:_ inflamed forearm tendon ("tennis elbow")

    3. _Torticollis:_ shortening of the neck muscle (sternocleido-mastoid)

    4. _Muscular dystrophy:_ wasting disease of the skeletal muscles

    5. _Bursitis:_ inflammation of the bursa, the fluid-filled sac that reduces friction as the joints move

D. Diagnostics and procedures

    1. _Manipulation_

        a. Skillful, dextrous treatment by hand

        b. Method of examination

        c. _ROM (range of motion):_ range, measured in degrees, in which a joint can be extended and flexed

        d. _PT (physical therapy):_ passive movement of a joint beyond its active limit of motion

    2. _X-ray:_ pictures of the muscle to see abnormalities

    3. _Goniometry:_ measurement of the flexion of a muscle

IV. DIGESTIVE SYSTEM

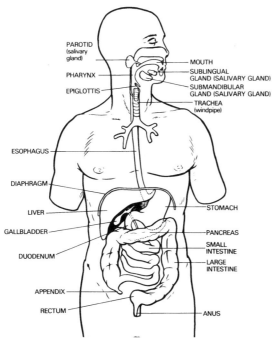

Figure 2-4 The digestive system.

For conditions of the digestive system, one would see a gastroenterologist.

A. Anatomy

1. _Mouth:_ where digestion starts
2. _Pharynx:_ passageway from nose and mouth to larynx and esophagus
3. _Esophagus:_ tube connecting the mouth and stomach
4. _Stomach:_ storage and digestive area for food
5. _Small intestines_
   a. _Duodenum:_ connected to the stomach by the pylorus; the first part of the small intestine
   b. _Jejunum:_ second part of the small intestine
   c. _Ileum:_ last portion of the small intestine
6. _Large intestines_
   a. _Cecum:_ blind pouch at the beginning of the large intestine; the lower portion is the appendix
   b. _Ascending colon_
   c. _Transverse colon_
   d. _Descending colon_
   e. _Sigmoid colon_
   f. _Rectum_
   g. _Anus_
7. _Liver_
   a. Glycogen storer, protein manufacturer, storer of vitamin B12, and of vitamins A, D, E, K, lipid metabolizer, cholesterol manufacturer, blood volume regulator, heparin source, clotting constituent source, bile secretor, detoxifier, and biotransformer of drugs
8. _Gallbladder_
   a. Releases bile into the small intestine for digestive aid
   b. Stores and concentrates bile from the liver
9. _Pancreas_
   a. _Exocrine part:_ produces pancreatic juices for digestion
   b. _Endocrine part:_ secretes insulin and glucagon directly into the bloodstream
10. _Appendix_
    a. Attachment at the first portion of the large intestine (cecum)
    b. _McBurney's point:_ site of tenderness associated with appendicitis
11. _Peritoneal membrane_
    a. Membrane surrounding the abdominal organs (not to be confused with the perineum, the area between the scrotum and anus in the male and the vulva and anus in the female)
12. _Visceral membranes:_ cover organs
13. _Parietal membranes:_ line cavities

B. Physiology
   1. Enzymes, acids, and muscle contractions break foods down for digestion
   2. *Peristalsis:* movement of food through the digestive system
C. Diseases and conditions
   1. *Crohn's disease:* inflammation of the GI tract, usually the small intestine
   2. *Cirrhosis:* chronic liver cell destruction
   3. *Hepatitis:* inflamed liver; skin may be jaundiced
   4. *Colitis:* inflammation of the colon
   5. *Gastroenteritis:* inflamed stomach and intestines
   6. *Hemorrhoids:* dilated, inflamed veins of the rectal mucosa
   7. *Ulcers:* eating away of the mucous membrane lining
   8. *Pyloric stenosis:* narrowing of the pyloric sphincter, which may prevent emptying of the contents of the stomach into the duodenum
   9. *Intussusception:* the telescoping or sliding of one part of the intestine into another
   10. *Hernia:* protruding of an organ through the wall of the cavity that contains it
       a. *Hiatal hernia:* stomach protruding upward into the mediastinal cavity
   11. *Esophagitis:* inflammation of the esophagus caused by acid reflux
D. Diagnostics and procedures
   1. *Cholecystography:* gallbladder x-ray
   2. *Upper GI:* barium swallow to x-ray upper GI tract
   3. *Lower GI:* barium enema to x-ray lower GI tract
   4. *Colonoscopy, sigmoidoscopy, gastroscopy, proctoscopy:* viewing into specific areas of the GI tract to detect problems
   5. *Hemorrhoidectomy:* excision of hemorrhoids

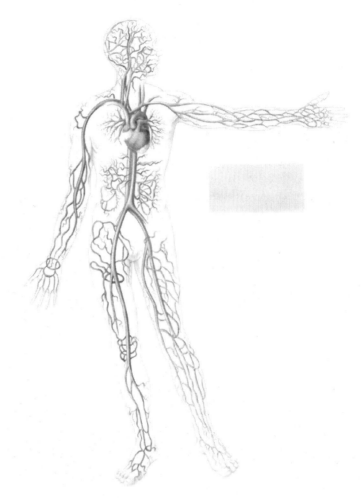

Figure 2-5 The cardiovascular system.

For diseases of the heart, one would visit a cardiologist or an internist.
  A. Anatomy and physiology
    1. *Heart:* pumps blood to all parts of the body
      a. *Sinoatrial node (SA node):* heart's pacemaker
      b. *Right atrium:* tricuspid valve; right ventricle
      c. *Left atrium:* bicuspid or mitral valve; left ventricle
          (largest chamber because of pumping action)

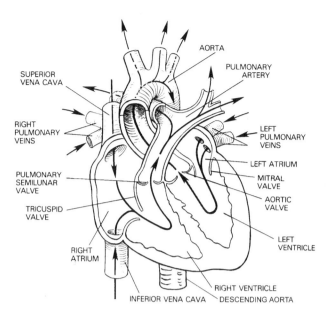

Figure 2-6 The heart.

2. *Arteries:* pulsate; carry blood away from the heart
   a. *Aorta:* main trunk of the arterial system; largest artery in the body
   b. *Carotid:* in the neck; check adult pulse here in CPR
   c. *Brachial:* check blood pressure here (located inside arm bend at the elbow)
   d. *Radial:* check pulse here (located inside the wrist area on the thumb side)
   e. *Femoral:* inner side of the femur; upper e r and groin area
3. *Veins:* have valves to resist backflow; carry blood back to the heart; appear dark blue
   a. *Vena cava:* principal vein draining the upper and lower portions of the body
   b. *Median cephalic:* venipuncture vein in the middle inner arm region (inside elbow bend)
4. *Capillaries:* connect arteries and veins; for food and oxygen exchange
5. *Blood components:* most blood cells are made in the red bone marrow
   a. *Red blood cells (erythrocytes)*
      • No nucleus
      • Biconcave
      • Contain hemoglobin; carry oxygen
      • Average count: 5,000,000 per cubic millimeter
      • Life span: 120 days
   b. *White blood cells (leukocytes)*
      • *Agranulocytes:* lymphocytes and monocytes (mononuclear)

- Granulocytes ("polys"): neutrophils, basophils, and eosinophils (polynuclear or multilobed)
- Combat infections
- Average count: 5,000 to 10,000 per cubic millimeter

c. *Platelets (thrombocytes)*
- Blood clotters
- Average count: 200,000 to 300,000 per cubic millimeter

d. *Plasma:* liquid portion of the blood
e. *Serum:* fluid portion of the blood after coagulation

6. *Spleen*
   a. Production of lymphocytes
   b. Storage of red blood cells
   c. Removal of old red blood cells

7. *Lymph system:* absorbs fluid and other substances for return to the circulatory system
   a. *Lymph nodes:* lymphoid tissue along the lymph system for filtering noxious substances from the body

B. Diseases and conditions
   1. *Tachycardia:* fast rhythm more than 100 beats/minute
   2. *Bradycardia:* slow rhythm less than 60 beats/minute
   3. *Heart block:* interruption of messages from the SA node to the atrioventricular node (AV node)
   4. *Anemia:* lack of certain elements in the blood
   5. *Angina pectoris:* spasm of the heart muscle because of decreased oxygen to the myocardium, causing pain and later ischemia; usually results from stress or physical activity
   6. *Arteriosclerosis:* hardening of the arteries
   7. *Atherosclerosis:* reduction of blood flow to the heart muscle in the myocardium because of buildup of fatty plaques in the coronary arteries, the arteries that supply the heart muscle
   8. *CVA (cerebrovascular accident):* commonly known as stroke
   9. *CHF (congestive heart failure):* decreased performance of the heart's pumping action
   10. *Hypertension:* elevated blood pressure; usually over 140/90
   11. *MI (myocardial infarction) or heart attack:* occlusion of the heart vessels causing deoxygenation and destruction of heart muscle
   12. *Rheumatic heart disease:* may follow upper respiratory strep infection, causing damage to the lining of the heart and the heart valves; with mitral valve problems, patient may need prophylactic penicillin prior to surgery and dental work
   13. *Mononucleosis:* increased mononuclear leukocytes in the blood; caused by Epstein-Barr virus

C. Diagnostics and procedures
   1. *EKG/ECG (electrocardiogram):* tracing of the heart's rhythm
   2. *Arteriogram:* x-ray of arteries

3. *Venogram:* x-ray of veins
4. *Cardiac catheterization:* visualizes heart activity and measures pressures within the heart's chambers
5. *Stress testing:* measures heart activity under controlled physical activity

VI. RESPIRATORY SYSTEM

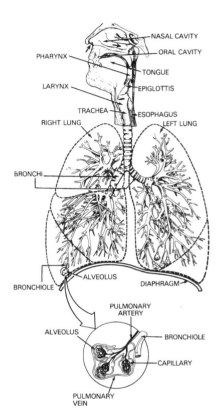

Figure 2-7 The respiratory system

For diseases of the respiratory system, one would visit a pulmonary or thoracic specialist or an internist.

A. Anatomy

1. *Nose:* air first enters here
2. *Larynx:* voice box
3. *Trachea (windpipe):* connects mouth and nose to the lungs
4. *Lungs:* consist of bronchi, bronchioles, and alveoli; where exchange of oxygen and carbon dioxide takes place
5. *Alveoli:* small air sacs in the lungs where carbon dioxide and oxygen exchange occurs
6. *Pleura:* serous membrane covering the lungs; has surfactant to lower surface tension

B. Physiology

1. *Exhalation:* breathing out
2. *Inhalation:* breathing in; external intercostal muscles assist with inspiration

3. Respirations are controlled by the medulla oblongata in the brain
4. Contractions of the diaphragm and accessory muscles cause inhalation and exhalation

C. Diseases and conditions
1. _Rhinitis:_ inflammation of the nose with sneezing, watery eyes, and nasal drip
2. _Asthma:_ chronic, usually allergic or infectious disorder that narrows air passages because of bronchospasms, causing wheezing or possibly severe dyspnea
3. _Bronchitis:_ inflammation of the bronchi caused by narrowed bronchial airways; usually patient has cough and shortness of breath
4. _Emphysema:_ enlargement of air spaces in the lungs, making exhalation difficult; usually with chronic cough and shortness of breath
5. _Pneumonia:_ acute infection of lung tissue
6. _TB (tuberculosis):_ infection causing nodules in the lungs

D. Diagnostics and procedures
1. _Pulmonary function tests using the spirometer:_ measure various lung capacities
2. _Bronchoscopy:_ viewing of the tissues of the lungs
3. _Chest x-ray:_ radiological picture of the lungs

VII. NERVOUS SYSTEM/SPECIAL SENSES
For diseases of the nervous system, one would visit a neurologist.

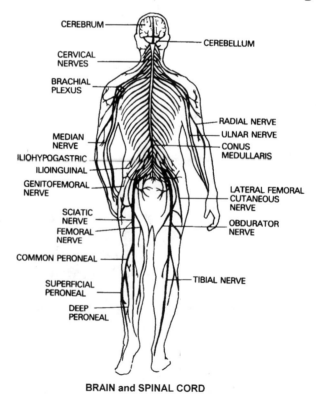

BRAIN and SPINAL CORD

Figure 2-8 The nervous system.

A. Anatomy
1. Peripheral nervous system and spine
   a. *Cranial nerves:* twelve pairs
      - *Olfactory:* sense of smell
      - *Optic:* vision
      - *Oculomotor:* eye movements, accommodation, and sensory perception
      - *Trochlear:* muscle sense and eye movement
      - *Trigeminal:* sensory perception for parts of the eye, nose, forehead, cheek, chin, and so on
      - *Abducens:* eye motion (problems with the abducens nerve = diplopia)
      - *Facial:* expressions of the face, taste (problems with the facial nerve = Bell's palsy)
      - *Vestibulocochlear (auditory, acoustic):* hearing and equilibrium
      - *Glossopharyngeal:* taste, swallowing
      - *Vagus:* coughing, sneezing, swallowing, hunger, and peristalsis
      - *Accessory:* neck muscle movement
      - *Hypoglossal:* tongue movements
   b. *Motor (movement) and sensory (senses) nerves*
      - *Neuron:* basic functioning unit of a nerve
      - *Synapse:* junction of neurons
   c. *Autonomic nervous system:* controls involuntary functions such as heartbeat, breathing, and digestion
      - *Sympathetic:* speeds up involuntary muscle action
      - *Parasympathetic:* slows down involuntary muscle action
   d. *Meninges:* covering that protects the spinal cord and brain
   e. *Cerebrospinal fluid:* cushions the brain and spinal cord, and provides nutrients; an important part of pressure regulation in the brain

2. Central nervous system

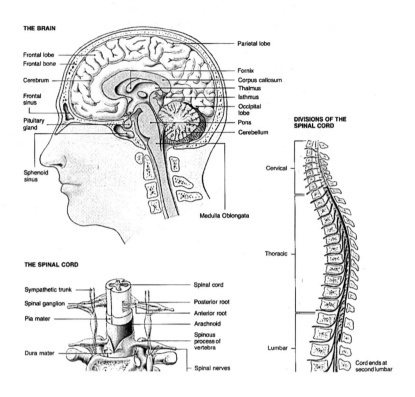

Figure 2-9 The brain and the spinal cord.

a. Brain
   - *Cerebrum:* largest area; sensory and motor activity; intellect
   - *Cerebellum:* smooth muscle movement and coordination
   - *Medulla oblongata:* vital control center influencing heartbeat, breathing, and temperature
   - *Pons:* influences breathing and is a reflex center
   - *Midbrain:* reflex center
   - *Hypothalmus:* regulates hormones, controls temperature, is the waking center, and controls appetite and sex drive
   - *Convolutions (gyri):* folds in the brain

B. Physiology
   1. Controls voluntary and involuntary functions, emotions, intellect, and senses

C. Diseases and conditions
   1. *Encephalitis:* severe inflammation of the brain
   2. *Meningitis:* inflammation of the covering of the brain and spinal cord
   3. *Hydrocephalus:* excessive fluid within the brain
   4. *Cerebral palsy:* brain damage before or during birth resulting in spasticity, underdevelopment, seizures, or mental retardation
   5. *Herpes zoster (shingles):* inflammation along a nerve caused by the varicella virus
   6. *Multiple sclerosis:* destruction of the myelin sheath, causing episodic tremors, weakness, mood swings, and vision changes
D. Diagnostics and procedures
   1. *CAT scan of the brain (computerized axial tomography):* x-rays of the layers of the brain
   2. *EEG (electroencephalogram):* recording of the brain waves
   3. *MRI of the brain (magnetic resonance imaging):* pictures of the brain using magnetic waves
   4. *Skull series:* x-rays of the brain
   5. *Lumbar puncture:* cerebrospinal fluid is aspirated for examination
E. Senses
   1. Eye

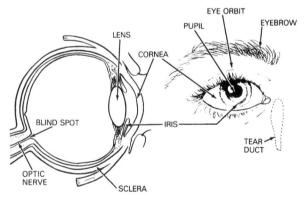

Figure 2-10 The eye.

   a. *Iris:* colored part of the eye
   b. *Pupil:* opening that constricts or dilates
   c. *Cornea:* transparent covering of the anterior part of the eye
   d. *Retina:* where an image focuses; inner layer of the eye
   e. *Conjunctiva:* transparent covering lining the eyelids and covering the eyeball
   f. *Sclera:* white, outer layer of the eye, just under the conjunctiva
   g. *Choroid:* middle, vascular layer of the inside of the eye

h. Disorders
- *Myopia:* ability to see near objects; nearsightedness
- *Hyperopia:* ability to see far objects; farsightedness
- *Presbyopia:* loss of accommodation (ability to adjust near to far, and far to near) due to age
- *Cataract:* cloudiness of the lens
- *Glaucoma:* increased pressure on the optic nerve inside the eye; checked by using a tonometer
- *Conjunctivitis:* inflamed lining of the lids

i. Diagnostics and procedures
- *Refraction:* checking for visual correction or glasses
- *Tonometry:* measuring intraocular pressure to check for glaucoma
- *Visual acuity:* evaluating distance vision using the Snellen eye chart or evaluating near vision using the near vision acuity chart or often, any type of everyday reading material, such as a telephone book and newspaper
- *Ishahara method:* checking color vision
- *Corneal transplants*

2. Ear

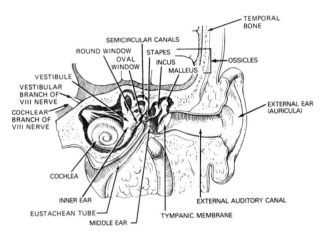

Figure 2-11 The ear.

a. *Tympanic membrane:* eardrum
b. *Middle ear:* malleus, incus, stapes (bones that conduct sound)
c. *Eustacian tube:* connects the ear to the throat (transfer of infections from the nose and throat to the ears occurs here; as children grow, this tube slants, resulting in less transfer of infection)
d. *Inner ear (cochlea):* contains sensory nerves for hearing and semicircular canals for balance
e. Disorders
- *Cerumen (wax) obstruction*
- *Otitis externa (swimmer's ear):* infection of the outer ear or otitis media (middle ear infection)

- *Méniere's disease:* dizziness (vertigo), tinnitus (ringing), and nerve loss
- *Otosclerosis:* hardening of the stapes
  f. Diagnostics and procedures
    - *Audiometry:* evaluation of hearing
    - *Myringotomy:* incision of the tympanic membrane

VIII. URINARY SYSTEM

For diseases of the urinary tract or problems with the male reproductive system one would see a urologist.

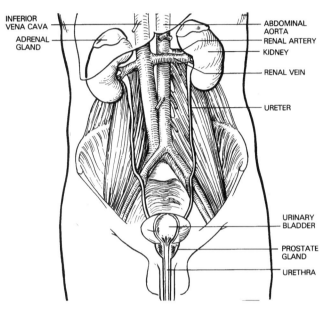

Figure 2-12 The urinary system.

A. Anatomy
  1. *Kidneys* (two)
     a. *Nephron:* most of the work is done here
     b. *Glomerulus:* filterer
     c. *Collecting tubules:* urine is concentrated here
     d. *Renal pelvis:* holding basin for urine until passage into the ureters
  2. *Ureters:* one per kidney, connecting the kidney to the bladder
  3. *Bladder:* reservoir for urine
  4. *Urethra:* tube leading from the bladder to the outside.
B. Physiology
  1. Urinary system serves to filter wastes from the body and eliminate them in the form of urine
C. Diseases and conditions
  1. *Cystitis:* Inflammation of the bladder
  2. *Glomerulonephritis:* inflammation of the glomerulus or filterer of the kidney

3. _Renal failure:_ cessation of kidney function
4. _Renal calculi (kidney stones):_ stone mass or masses present in the pelvis of the kidney
5. _Incontinence:_ inability to retain urine (or feces) because of loss of muscle sphincter control.

D. Diagnostics and procedures
1. _Cystoscopy:_ viewing of the bladder
2. _Urinalysis and 24-hour collections:_ analysis of the urine physically and chemically or collection to check the amount of output
3. _IVP (intravenous pyelography):_ x-rays of the urinary tract
4. _Dialysis:_ mechanical removal of waste products from the blood
5. _Transplants:_ replacement of a nonfunctioning kidney with a kidney from a donor

IX. REPRODUCTIVE SYSTEM

For problems of the female reproductive system, one would see a gynecologist; if pregnant, an obstetrician. The male would see a urologist.

A. Female anatomy

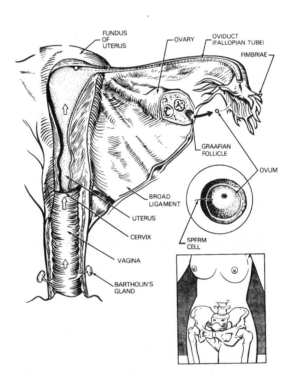

Figure 2-13 The female reproductive system.

1. _Ovaries (two):_ primary reproductive organs
2. _Fallopian tubes:_ next to the ovaries and connecting to the uterus
3. _Uterus:_ normally hollow muscular organ
   a. _Cervix:_ the lower opening into the uterus

4. _Vagina:_ opening from the outside of body connecting to the cervix
5. _Breasts:_ mammary glands

B. Male anatomy

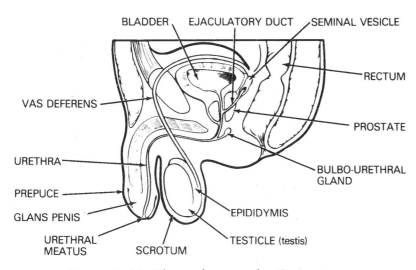

BLADDER   EJACULATORY DUCT   SEMINAL VESICLE

RECTUM

VAS DEFERENS

PROSTATE

URETHRA

BULBO-URETHRAL
GLAND

PREPUCE

GLANS PENIS

EPIDIDYMIS

URETHRAL
MEATUS   SCROTUM   TESTICLE (testis)

Figure 2-14 The male reproductive system.

1. _Testes:_ primary sex organs of the male; suspended in the scrotum
2. _Penis:_ male organ of copulation/urination
3. _Prostate gland:_ muscular secreting tissue surrounding the urethra

C. Female physiology

1. _Ovaries:_ for development of eggs or ova and estrogen secretion
2. _Uterine lining or endometrium:_ builds up to prepare for implantation of fertilized ovum or for shedding, as in menstruation
3. _Breasts:_ for milk production

D. Male physiology

1. _Testes:_ produce sperm and secrete testosterone
2. _Penis:_ has within it the urethra, a tube for expelling semen or urine
3. _Prostate:_ contracts during ejaculation and secretes part of the seminal fluid

E. Diseases and conditions

1. _Hydrocele:_ excessive fluid in the scrotum of the male
2. _Prostatic hypertrophy:_ enlargement of the prostate gland
3. _Prostatectomy:_ excision of the prostate gland
4. _Endometriosis:_ endometrium-like tissue found in abnormal places, usually the pelvic area
5. _Hysterectomy:_ cutting out of the uterus
6. _Mastectomy:_ removal of the breast due to cancer

7. _STD (sexually transmitted diseases):_ AIDS, syphillis, gonorrhea, chlamydial infections, trichomoniasis, genital herpes
8. _Ectopic pregnancy:_ implantation of a fertilized ova somewhere other than the uterus, usually the fallopian tubes
9. _Prostatitis:_ inflammation of the prostate gland
10. _Vaginitis:_ inflammation of the vagina caused by yeast, bacteria, or other organisms
11. _Impotence:_ inability to achieve or maintain erection of the penis

F. Diagnostics and procedures
1. Testicular self-examination
   a. Testicles rolled gently between thumb and forefingers of both hands
   b. Lumps or knots reported to a doctor
2. Breast self-examination
   a. Breasts rubbed in shower with flat fingers (not fingertips) to feel for lumps (circling breasts, inside out)
   b. Reflection in mirror: hands by side, then over head; look for asymmetry, dimpling, swelling, or nipple changes
   c. Supine: circle breasts inside out again with flat fingers; check nipples for discharge by gently squeezing
3. _Pap smear:_ obtaining microscopic samples of the cervical area to check for abnormal cells
4. _Mammogram:_ x-ray of the breasts
5. _D and C (dilation and curettage):_ scraping of the inside of the uterus
6. _Cryotherapy or cauterization:_ freeze or burn therapy
7. _Amniocentesis:_ puncture of the amniotic sac to remove fluid for study

X. ENDOCRINE SYSTEM
For diseases of the endocrine system, one would see an endocrinologist.

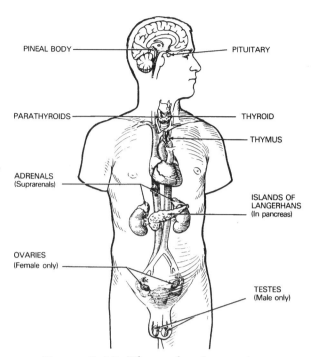

Figure 2-15 The endocrine system.

A. Anatomy
1. *Pituitary gland:* located at the base of the brain (called "master gland")
   a. Anterior lobe hormones
      • Growth hormone
      • Prolactin
      • Thyroid-stimulating hormone
      • Adrenocorticotropic hormone
      • Follicle-stimulating hormone
   b. Posterior lobe hormones
      • Antidiuretic hormone
      • Oxytocin
2. *Thyroid gland:* located in the anterior part of the neck
   a. Thyroxine
   b. Triiodothyronine
   c. Calcitonin
3. *Adrenal gland:* located at the top of each kidney
   a. Adrenal medulla hormones
      • Epinephrine
      • Norepinephrine
   b. Adrenal cortex hormones
      • Aldosterone
      • Glucocorticoids/cortisol
      • Androgens or sex hormones

4. _Parathyroid:_ located on the posterior surface of the thyroid gland
   a. Parathormone
5. _Pancreas:_ located behind the stomach
   a. Islets (Islands) of Langerhans
      - Insulin
      - Glucagon
6. _Pineal gland:_ located in third ventricle of the brain
   a. Melatonin
7. _Thymus:_ located behind the sternum
   a. Thymosin
8. _Reproductive glands_
   a. _Ovaries:_ located in the female pelvis
      - Estrogen
      - Progesterone
   b. _Testes:_ located in the male scrotum
      - Testosterone

B. Physiology

1. _Pituitary:_ secretions controlled by the hypothalmus
   a. _Growth hormone:_ stimulates cell growth and reproduction
   b. _Prolactin:_ promotes female breast development and milk production and stimulates male sex hormone production
   c. _Thyroid-stimulating hormone:_ controls secretion of the thyroid gland's hormones
   d. _Adrenocorticotropic hormone:_ controls secretion of certain hormones from the adrenal cortex
   e. _Follicle-stimulating hormone:_ influences the reproductive organs
   f. _Antidiuretic hormone:_ reduces excretion of the kidneys, sometimes affects blood pressure
   g. _Oxytocin:_ causes uterine contractions and influences milk production
2. _Thyroid:_ removes iodine from the blood
   a. _Thyroxine and triiodothyronine:_ influences metabolism, protein synthesis, and maturation of the nervous system
   b. _Calcitonin:_ decreases blood calcium and phosphate levels
3. _Adrenals_
   a. _Epinephrine:_ like sympathetic nervous system, increases heart rate; is a vasoconstrictor and thus increases blood pressure; is a bronchiole relaxer
   b. _Aldosterone:_ helps conserve sodium and water in the kidneys and decreases potassium reabsorption
   c. _Glucocorticoids:_ influence protein, fat, and glucose metabolism, therefore influencing blood glucose; also serve as antiinflammatories

      d. *Sex hormones:* promote sex characteristics and functions

  4. *Parathyroid glands*

      a. *Parathormone:* increases blood calcium and decreases blood phosphate

  5. *Pancreas*

      a. *Insulin:* increases metabolism of carbohydrates; decreases blood sugar

      b. *Glucagon:* stimulates release of glycogen from the liver promoting increased blood sugar

  6. *Pineal*

      a. *Melatonin:* appears to decrease reproductive activities by inhibiting gonadotropic hormones

  7. *Thymus*

      a. *Thymosin:* affects lymphocyte production

  8. *Reproductive glands*

      a. *Estrogen, progesterone and testosterone:* promote sexual characteristics and functions

C. Diseases and conditions

  1. *Dwarfism:* lack of growth hormone; if during childhood, called cretinism

  2. *Gigantism:* excess of growth hormone in childhood

  3. *Acromegaly:* excess of growth hormone in adulthood

  4. *Hypothyroidism:* decrease in thyroid hormone production, and thus a decrease in metabolic rate; called myxedema in adulthood

  5. *Hyperthyroidism:* excess of thyroid hormone production, and thus an increase in metabolic rate; Graves' disease

      a. *Exophthalmia:* bulging eyes

      b. *Goiter:* enlarged thyroid gland because of a lack of iodine

  6. *Tetany:* uncontrolled twitching of the muscles because of hypoparathyroidism

  7. *Cushing's disease:* excess of glucocorticoids causing edema of the face and fatty tissue on the back ("moonface" and "buffalo hump")

  8. *Diabetes mellitus:* high blood sugar and sugar in the urine because of a lack of insulin

D. Diagnostics and procedures

  1. *Thyroidectomy:* surgical removal of the thyroid gland

  2. *Thyroid function tests:* check function of the thyroid gland

  3. *Thyroid scan:* checks thyroid's absorption ability

  4. *Glucose tolerance test:* checks patient's metabolism of glucose; confirmatory test for diabetes

1. The longest and strongest bone is the:
   a. ilium
   b. spine
   c. femur
   d. humerus

2. The calcaneus is closest to the:
   a. carpals
   b. clavicle
   c. patella
   d. tarsals

3. A cervical fracture can occur only in:
   a. C-5
   b. C-8
   c. C-10
   d. C-12

4. Muscles that move food along the digestive tract are:
   a. striated
   b. under conscious control
   c. voluntary
   d. smooth

5. What is the correct sequence of food movement through the small intestine?
   a. duodenum, jejunum, ileum
   b. jejunum, ileum, duodenum
   c. duodenum, ileum, jejunum
   d. ileum, duodenum, jejunum

6. The pyloric orifice is the opening between the:
   a. esophagus and stomach
   b. rectum and anus
   c. duodenum and stomach
   d. mouth and trachea

7. The largest part of the brain, which also controls higher mental faculties, is the:
   a. cerebrum
   b. cerebellum
   c. cerumen
   d. medulla oblongata

8. The valve between the left atrium and left ventricle is the:
   a. mitral valve
   b. tricuspid valve
   c. semilunar valve
   d. coronary valve

9. The normal pacemaker of the heart is the:
   a. AV node
   b. EKG
   c. bundle of His
   d. SA node

10. Most of the work done by the kidney is done by the:
    a. urethra
    b. renal pelvis
    c. nephron units
    d. ureters

11. Oxytocin is responsible for:
    a. conservation of sodium in the kidney
    b. lactation and uterine contractions in labor
    c. secretion of the growth hormone
    d. Cushing's syndrome

12. The artery site for taking blood pressure is the:
    a. carotid
    b. temporal
    c. dorsalis pedis
    d. brachial

13. Sebum is produced by the:
    a. sweat gland
    b. sudoriforous gland
    c. sebaceous gland
    d. pineal gland

14. A fungus affecting the scalp, feet, or body is:
    a. vitiligo
    b. ringworm
    c. psoriasis
    d. urticaria

15. Broken bones that puncture the skin are called:
    a. compound fractures
    b. simple fractures
    c. impacted fractures
    d. comminuted fractures

16. Vital capacity or the amount of air the lungs can hold is measured by:
    a. bronchoscopy
    b. pneumograms
    c. spirometry
    d. respirometer

17. Color vision is usually checked by the:
    a. Snellen chart
    b. tonometer
    c. slit lamp
    d. Ishahara method

18. Ectopic pregnancies are usually located in the:
    a. ovaries
    b. uterus
    c. endometrium
    d. fallopian tubes

19. Which glandular secretion mimics the sympathetic nervous system?
    a. growth hormone
    b. epinephrine
    c. calcitonin
    d. estrogen

20. Which glandular secretion reduces blood sugar levels?
    a. insulin
    b. glucagon
    c. testosterone
    d. prolactin

Answers

1. c Femur, the upper leg bone. The ilium is one of the wide bones of the pelvis. A spine is a sharp process of bone; the spinal column is composed of 33 vertebrae or small bones. The humerus is the upper arm bone and is shorter than the femur.

2. d The calcaneus is the heel bone of the foot, which is closest to the tarsals in the foot. The carpals are the wrist bones. The clavicle is the anterior shoulder bone. The patella is the knee bone.

3. a C-5. There are seven cervical vertebrae. C-5 can be fractured, but there are no such vertebrae as C-8, C-10, or C-12.

4. d Smooth muscles, which are involuntary and not under conscious control. Striated muscles are skeletal muscles for movement and are voluntary and under conscious control.

5. a The stomach contents empty through the pyloric sphincter into the duodenum. From the duodenum, the contents are moved by peristalsis through the jejunum and into the ileum.

6. c Duodenum and stomach. The rectum connects directly into the anus. The esophagus connects directly into the stomach. The mouth leads into the esophagus.

7. a The cerebrum, which controls sensory and motor activity, conscious thought, and intellect. The cerebellum controls coordination and smooth muscle movement. Cerumen is ear wax. The medulla oblongata influences heartbeat, breathing, and temperature.

8. a Mitral valve. The tricuspid valve is between the right atrium and the right ventricle. The semilunar valve is between the right ventricle and the pulmonary artery. There is no such valve as the coronary valve.

9. d The sinoatrial node is the heart's pacemaker. The AV (atrioventricular) node and the bundle of His also carry impulses along the nerve fibers but do not initiate impulses as the SA node does. The EKG is a diagnostic tool to check the rhythm of the heart.

10. c The nephron units are where tubes and filters act to remove wastes from the blood. The ureters are tubes leading from the kidneys to the bladder. The urethra leads from the bladder to the outside of the body. The renal pelvis is a holding tank for the urine before it enters the ureter.

11. b Lactation and uterine contractions in labor. Aldosterone promotes conservation of sodium and excretion of potassium in the kidney. Secretion of the growth hormone is controlled by a growth hormone-releasing hormone from the hypothalmus. Cushing's syndrome is caused by hyperproduction of the glucocorticoids of the adrenal glands.

12. d Brachial, which is located in the inner bend of the arm. Blood pressure would not be taken in the carotid, which is in the neck, or the temporal, which is between the ear and eye, or the dorsalis pedis, which is above the foot.

13. c Sebaceous gland. Sweat glands and sudoriforous glands are the same and they produce sweat or sudor. The pineal gland produces melatonin.

14. b Ringworm is a known fungal infection. Vitiligo and psoriasis are not known to be fungal. Urticaria is usually caused by an allergen.

15. a Compound fractures. A simple fracture does not penetrate the skin. The ends of the bones in an impacted fracture penetrate each other. A comminuted fracture breaks into little pieces.

16. c Spirometry. Bronchoscopy is a viewing into the lungs. A pneumogram is a record of respiratory movements. A respirometer evaluates the character of respirations.

17. d The Ishahara method, which illustrates colored dots shaped into numbers with surrounding dots of a different color. The Snellen chart is used to measure distance visual acuity. The tonometer measures eye pressure. The slit lamp is used to look at and magnify the eye.

18. d Ectopic pregnancies can be anywhere outside the uterus but usually implant in the fallopian tubes.

19. b Epinephrine mimics the sympathetic nervous system in that it speeds heart rate, increases blood pressure, and relaxes bronchioles. Growth hormone increases size and reproduction of cells. Calcitonin lowers blood levels of calcium and phosphate. Estrogen stimulates secondary sex characteristics.

20. a Insulin. Glucagon increases blood sugar. Testosterone is a male sex hormone that stimulates secondary sex characteristics. Prolactin promotes breast development and milk production.

3

Professionalism

CHAPTER OUTLINE

Professional Behavior and Traits
Job Description
Professional Organizations
Continuing Education
Ethics
Quality Assurance and Risk Management

I. PROFESSIONAL BEHAVIOR AND TRAITS
  A. Desirable qualities
    1. Intelligence
    2. Friendliness
    3. Empathy
    4. Punctuality
    5. Maintainence of good health and hygiene
    6. Membership in professional organizations
    7. Currency of knowledge and continued reading of literature pertaining to the field of medical assisting
    8. Knowledge of the scope of practice and the limitations of practice within that scope
    9. Cooperative team membership
    10. Maintenance of poise and self-control
    11. Self-motivation
    12. Good attitude and positive outlook
    13. No use of profanity
    14. No gum chewing
    15. Good English usage and good communication skills
  B. Professional dress
    1. Conservative and business-like
    2. Conservative necklines and hemlines
    3. Clean, wrinkle-free, and polished
    4. Clean breath and clean smell (remember that some people are allergic to perfumes)
    5. Overall neatness

II. JOB DESCRIPTION
  A. Medical assistant
    1. Professional and multiskilled
    2. Dedicated to assisting in all aspects of medical practice under a physician
    3. Patient caregiver
    4. Skilled in clinical, administrative, and laboratory procedures
    5. Capable at managerial and supervisory roles
    6. Has good communication skills
    7. Adheres to ethical and legal practices
    8. Skilled in emergency management

III. PROFESSIONAL ORGANIZATIONS
Membership is a must!
  A. *AAMA:* American Association of Medical Assistants
    1. Journal: *The Professional Medical Assistant* or *PMA*
    2. Certification awarded to those passing the national examination

    3. Recertification every five years; 60 recertification points needed (20 general, 20 administrative, and 20 clinical)
    4. Local AAMA chapter membership and state MA society membership when joining national organization
       a. Continuing education by attending meetings and seminars, study courses through AAMA or *PMA*, college courses, and authorship
  B. *AAMT:* American Association of Medical Transcriptionists
    1. Bimonthly newsletter and quarterly journal
    2. Voluntary certification by examination
    3. Recertification every three years; 30 CEUs needed
  C. *RMA:* Registered Medical Assistants
    1. Establishment by American Medical Technologists (AMT)
    2. Certification by examination
    3. Revalidation every five years
  D. *PSI:* Professional Secretaries International; *CPS:* certified professional secretary
    1. Examination and work requirements for certification
    2. Two-day examination twice a year

IV. CONTINUING EDUCATION

  A. CEUs (continuing education units) obtained in many ways
    1. Program credit at local, state, and national meetings
    2. Workshops approved by each organization
    3. Tests following articles in professional magazines
    4. Guided study programs through the mail

V. ETHICS

  A. AAMA Code of Ethics
    1. *Dignity of the patient:* maintained with all patients regardless of circumstances
    2. *Confidentiality:* practiced in all areas concerning patients
    3. *Professionalism:* practiced at all times
    4. *Continuing education:* pursued for professional growth
    5. *Good citizenship:* observed by participation in community affairs

VI. QUALITY ASSURANCE AND RISK MANAGEMENT

  A. Monitoring and evaluating systems in place
  B. Standards of quality established and practiced
  C. Accreditation of all areas utilized for continued self-assessment
  D. Safety promotion in all areas; risks identified and reduced
  E. Lack of quality care or practices identified and improved
  F. Liabilities reduced; liability insurance in needed areas

QUESTIONS

1. The journal for the AAMA is the ___PMA___.

2. Four professional organizations a medical assistant might join are _AAMA_, _RMA_, _AAMt_, and _PSI_.

3. CEU means _Continuing Education units_

4. How are CEUs earned?

5. Name five components of the AAMA code of ethics.

6. Explain risk management.

7. Explain quality assurance.

8. Describe a professional.

Answers

1. <u>The Professional Medical Assistant</u>

2. AAMA (American Association of Medical Assistants), RMA (Registered Medical Assistants), AAMT (American Association of Medical Transcriptionists), PSI (Professional Secretaries International)

3. Continuing education units

4. By attending local, state, and national AAMA workshops, attending organization approved workshops, testing after reading articles in professional magazines, and using home-study guided programs through the mail

5. Dignity of the patient, confidentiality, professionalism, continuing education, and good citizenship

6. Risk management is identifying all risks possible in a particular practice and following up with actions designed to prevent problems

7. Quality assurance is identifying standards of quality in a practice, taking measures to evaluate whether or not standards are met, and checking on any unmet standards to ensure improvement

8. A professional is one who acts as a professional (e.g., does not chew gum, or swear); has desirable qualities such as intelligence, friendliness, empathy, punctuality, positive outlook, and cheerful attitude; works as a team member, and has poise and self-control; looks professional, (e.g., wears conservative makeup, and clothes with neither plunging necklines nor very short hemlines); is clean, polished, polite, and uses good grammar; knows and practices within the scope of the profession and keeps abreast of changes

4

Patient Communication

CHAPTER OUTLINE

Behavioral Influences
Effective Techniques of Communication
Noneffective Communication
Body Language
Telephone Communication

I. BEHAVIORAL INFLUENCES
   A. *Maslow's hierarchy of needs:* one must fulfill one's own needs in order to relate to others and use one's talents to the fullest
      1. Physiological (thirst, hunger, sleep, sex)
      2. Safety
      3. Love and belonging
      4. Self-worth and esteem
      5. Self-actualization (reaching one's potential)
      6. Transcendence (spiritualism)
   B. *Elizabeth Kubler-Ross:* death and dying stages
      1. Denial (not me!)
      2. Anger (why me?)
      3. Bargaining
      4. Depression
      5. Acceptance
   C. *"Know thyself":* one must have self-knowledge to understand others
      1. Knowledge of own values
      2. Understanding of cultural differences
      3. Understanding of patients' perceptions of illness
         a. Loss of job due to illness may cause anxiety and anger
         b. Loss of independence due to illness may cause depression
      4. Defense mechanisms
         a. *Repression:* pushing unpleasant thoughts into unconsciousness
         b. *Displacement:* transferring of one's own feelings to another
         c. *Projection:* blaming another for one's own faults
         d. *Rationalization:* justification of behavior by giving acceptable reasons for behavior rather than the real reason
         e. *Withdrawal:* retreat from the painful situation
         f. *Malingering:* pretending to be ill to avoid unpleasant problems

II. EFFECTIVE TECHNIQUES OF COMMUNICATION
Sender-receiver feedback is essential!
   A. *Silent periods so that patient can voice feelings*
   B. *Good listening skills*
      1. Practice of active, involved listening
      2. Facial expressions to show acknowledgment of message heard
      3. Leaning of body toward person shows interest
      4. Head nodding encourages the speaker to continue

C. *Open-ended questions:* "Tell me about your pain," instead of "Does it hurt here?"

D. *No false reassurances:* "We'll do the best we can," not "Everything will be fine."

E. *Empathy:* putting oneself in another person's place to realize the other person's feelings

F. *Good eye contact*

G. *Repetition:* repeating what is said to be sure it was understood correctly (especially doctor's orders, phone numbers, order numbers, lab reports)

H. *Clarification and feedback* ("Do you mean...")

I. *Special cases:* all persons have self-worth; all persons are unique; treat all without judging

   1. *Deaf and elderly:* speak face to face in case they read lips; treat them as adults, have patience, and allow independent decision making

   2. *Children:* give directions in terms they can understand

   3. *Angry patients:* speak softly, take them to a private area, try to calm them down, and get to the bottom of the problem

   4. *Anxious patients:* give simple directions; give written directions; recognize and accept anxiety; listen to and acknowledge fears

   5. *Cultural differences:* may have to find alternative treatment if patient will not comply for cultural or religious reasons

   6. *Teenagers:* allow privacy; treat as adults

   7. *Dying patients:* acknowledge grief; listen to fears; give no false reassurances

III. NONEFFECTIVE COMMUNICATION

A. *Criticism and lecturing:* "You don't help your situation when you don't take your medicine."

B. *Preaching:* "Don't you know smoking is wrong?"

C. *False reassurances:* "Everything will be fine."

D. *Changing the subject:* "It sure is sunny today."

E. *Put-downs:* "You shouldn't be afraid of the doctor."

F. *Closed questions (questions answered by one word such as "yes" or "no"):* "Are you hurting?"

IV. BODY LANGUAGE

A. *Facial expression:* nonverbal behavior

   1. *Congruence:* verbal and nonverbal message should be the same for good communication

   2. Expressions should be nonjudgmental

   3. Eye contact should be maintained to show interest

B. *Touch:* can show sensitivity as long as receiver is accepting of touch

C. *Posture*
 1. *Standing straight:* promotes the idea of self-assurance
 2. *Slumped posture:* promotes the idea of depression, or lack of confidence
 3. *Arms crossed:* promotes an opinionated, unapproachable image
D. *Movements*
 1. *Drumming of the fingers:* boredom, impatience
 2. *Scratching the head:* puzzlement, confusion
 3. *Tapping the foot:* impatience
E. *Personal space*
 1. Shorter distances between people indicate more intimate communication
F. *Clothing and appearance:* send messages of professionalism or slovenliness
 1. *Professional:* crisp, clean white uniform
 2. *Nonprofessional:* shirttail out, hair uncombed, runs in hose, unkempt

V. TELEPHONE COMMUNICATION
A. First impression of the office; therefore, answer pleasantly
 1. Identity of office and of self (and caller)
B. Hold the receiver 2 to 3 inches from mouth
C. Types of calls received
 1. *Appointments*
 2. *Prescriptions*
 3. *Test results*
 4. *Emergencies:* may need to triage (prioritize according to most severe)
  a. High fevers
  b. Acute illnesses
  c. Medication allergies (possible anaphylaxis)
  d. Dehydration
 5. *Doctor's calls or referrals*
  a. Necessity to put through to the doctor right away, but try to have patient's chart in doctor's hand before connecting doctor to caller

1. The most basic needs in Maslow's Hierarchy of needs are:
   a. thirst, hunger, sleep, sex
   b. self-esteem
   c. to be loved and belong
   d. transcendence

2. The final stage in Elizabeth Kubler-Ross' death and dying stages is:
   a. denial
   b. acceptance
   c. anger
   d. bargaining

3. To pretend sickness to avoid an unpleasant situation is:
   a. withdrawal
   b. repression
   c. projection
   d. malingering

4. Effective techniques of communication include all but one of the following:
   a. silent periods
   b. open-ended questions
   c. false reassurances
   d. good listening

5. When answering the phone, say:
   a. "Good morning"
   b. "May I help you?"
   c. "Will you hold please?"
   d. the office name and your own name

6. Choose the best answer to the following statement: "When I die, I want you to come to my funeral."
   a. "You're not going to die."
   b. "The weather is too pretty to talk about dying."
   c. "What are you really saying, Mrs. Jones?"
   d. "Will they be serving chicken?"

Answers

1. a Maslow's Hirearchy of needs begins with the most basic needs of hunger, thirst, sleep, and sex. Second is the need for safety; third, the need for love and belonging; fourth, the need for self-esteem; fifth, the need for self-actualization; and last or at the top, is transcendence or spiritualism.

2. b Elizabeth Kubler-Ross' stages of death and dying are, from first to last, denial, anger, bargaining, depression, and acceptance.

3. d Malingering. Withdrawal is retreat from a painful situation. Projection is blaming another for one's own faults. Repression is pushing unpleasant thoughts into one's subconscience.

4. c Giving false reassurances is an ineffective communication technique. When you say everything is going to be all right, the patient may feel you are dismissing his/her worries as insignificant and may also lose trust in you when everything does not turn out all right. The rest are effective techniques in that silent periods give the patient a chance to collect his/her thoughts and reflect on what he/she is going to say; open-ended questions give the patient a chance to elaborate on a question rather than answer just yes or no; and good listening is always an effective form of communicating.

5. d The office name and your own name are musts when answering the telephone. The other answers are pleasantries but not necessities.

6. c "What are you really saying, Mrs. Jones?" is getting to the crux of the matter. You will get clarification of what Mrs. Jones really wants to say.

5

Medical Law

CHAPTER OUTLINE

Legal Terms
Malpractice Prevention
Physician Regulations
Medical Office Regulations

I. LEGAL TERMS

A. *Ethics:* relating to a set of moral values or actions

B. *Respondeat superior ("Let the master answer"):* doctrine which states that the employer is responsible for the actions of an employee

C. *Medical practice acts:* state statutes that define the practice of medicine

D. *Standard of care:* measurement requiring a doctor to use the ordinary, reasonable skill, experience, and knowledge used by other reputable physicians under the same or similar circumstances in caring for patients

E. *Contract:* agreement between two or more competent persons upon consideration or payment to do or not to do a specific activity

F. *Tort:* wrongful act of one person against another that causes harm to person or property.

G. *Agent:* a person representing or acting for another

H. *Arbitration:* procedure by which an impartial person, selected by the parties involved, resolves a dispute at a hearing

I. *Emancipated minor:* person under the age of 18 years who is financially independent

J. *False imprisonment:* detention against a person's will

K. *Invasion of privacy:* disclosure of a person's private affairs without prior consent

L. *Malpractice:* professional misconduct; lack of skill; wrongful practice that causes injury to the patient

M. *Negligence:* not doing an act that a prudent person would do, resulting in injury

N. *Four Ds of negligence:* duty, derelict, direct cause, damages

O. *Res ipsa loquitur ("the thing speaks for itself"):* doctrine where there is an inference of negligence due to the attendant circumstances, e.g., medical malpractice evidenced by a pair of scissors sewn up in a patient

P. *Privileged communication:* that which cannot be made public, as that which arises from the doctor–patient relationship

Q. *Statute of limitations:* specific period of time in which a lawsuit can be filed or initiated

R. *Subpoena duces tecum:* an order to provide records or documents to the court

S. *Locum tenens:* substitute or representative

T. *Liability:* obligation by law to pay or make amends for an act

U. *Scope of practice:* legal bounds within which a person practices her/his profession

V. *Quid pro quo:* the giving of something in return for something else

II. MALPRACTICE PREVENTION

A. Kindness to patients maintained: sincere caring for patients (generally, patients hate to sue people who have been sincerely kind and caring toward them)

B. Performance within the scope of practice

C. Compliance with state laws

D. Learned knowledge of safe and aseptic practice used

E. Documentation of all patient visits, calls and correspondence, missed appointments, and prescriptions authorized by telephone to the pharmacist

F. No telephone advice given

G. Patient data such as lab reports seen and initialed by doctor prior to filing

H. Confidentiality practiced

I. Cures never guaranteed

J. Explanations of appointment delays given along with apologies

K. Estimates of fees given with explanations that they are just estimates

L. Informed consents secured when needed along with documentation of the discussion held

M. Doctor informed of patient complaints

N. Documentation kept of discharge or release of patients and certified letter sent when withdrawing from a case

III. PHYSICIAN REGULATIONS

A. *Controlled Substances Act:* regulates dispensing of scheduled drugs

   1. *Registration with the DEA (Drug Enforcement Agency):* renewal every three years
   2. *Record keeping:* include patient given drug, drug, dosage, date given, and reason given; records kept two years
   3. *Inventory:* on date of registration and every two years following date of initial inventory
   4. *Drug schedules*
      a. *I:* highest potential for abuse; not legalized (marijuana)
      b. *II:* high abuse potential, but accepted medically; must use special DEA form in triplicate (quaalude, codeine, morphine, opium derivatives, stimulants, amphetamines)
      c. *III:* less abuse potential; may become dependent (amphetamine-like substances, narcotic drugs with limited amounts of codeine)
      d. *IV:* lower abuse potential (valium, minor tranquilizers)
      e. *V:* least potential for abuse (lomotil, drugs with limited amounts of narcotics)

5. Log of controlled drugs with patient name, drug, dosage , and date given
   a. *Patient's chart:* record of controlled drugs given should agree with log
   b. *Wasting of drugs:* log and have witness
B. *Physician licensure requirements*
   1. Legal age
   2. Moral character
   3. Completion of all educational requirements and passing of boards
   4. Renewal
      a. Periodically (usually yearly, with proof of 50 hours of CEUs)
   5. Revocation/suspension
      a. Conviction of crime
      b. Unprofessional conduct
      c. Personal or professional incapacity
C. *Uniform Anatomical Gift Act*
   1. Patient donation of body or parts of body after death for research or transplant
      a. Sound mind and legal age required
      b. No money exchange
      c. Time of death determined by a doctor having no interest in the transplant or research
D. *Living will*
   1. Patients elect not to receive life-sustaining measures if a life-threatening event takes place (must be decided prior to any life-threatening event)
      a. Competency of patient a must
      b. Two witnesses needed
E. *Medical practice acts:* define practices for physicians in each state
   1. Doctor must practice within the scope of his training and not beyond the limits of his state's medical practice acts
F. *Public health duties*
   1. Reports to proper authorities
      a. Vital statistics: birth, death, and fetal death
      b. Communicable diseases
      c. Known or suspected abuse
      d. Drug abuse
      e. Criminal acts
G. *Informed consent:* consent for an invasive procedure after the patient is informed of risks, the procedure itself, alternative treatments, and possible results if treatment is not performed. After patient signs an informed consent, it is appropriate to document in the patient's chart that questions were answered to the patient's satisfaction and a discussion of risks, alternative treatments, and so on, was held.

H. *Worker's compensation:* doctor must register with state workers' compensation boards yearly

IV. MEDICAL OFFICE REGULATIONS

A. *Truth-in-Lending Act, Regulation Z:* any bill paid in more than four installments must be written and an indication made as to whether or not interest will be charged

B. *CLIA (Clinical Laboratory Improvement Amendments):* medical office laboratories must follow certain regulations for quality assurance

C. *Hazardous wastes:* must be disposed of according to OSHA (Occupational Safety and Health Act) requirements

D. *Taxes:* federal, state, and local guidelines must be adhered to

   1. All new employees must fill out W-4 forms (employee's withholding allowance certificate)
   2. W-2 forms must be given by January 31 (wage and tax statements)
   3. *FICA:* Federal Insurance Contributions Act—Social Security taxes (employer and employee contribute)
      a. *OASI:* Old Age and Survivors Insurance
      b. *HI:* hospitalization under Medicare
      c. *DI:* disability insurance
   4. *FUTA:* Federal Unemployment Tax Act (employer contributions only)
   5. *Gross earnings:* amount actually made
   6. *Net earnings:* amount given employee after taxes and other deductions

E. *Release of patient information:* always need permission and signature of patient to release any medical information

F. *Sexual harassment:* Sexual discrimination that is gender-based; job advancement offered in exchange for sexual favors; inappropriate touching

QUESTIONS

1. Physicians are required to report which of the following:
   a. measles
   b. births and deaths
   c. child abuse
   d. all of the above

2. "Let the master answer" (the doctor is responsible for the acts of employees):
   a. locum tenens
   b. res ipsa loquitur
   c. respondeat superior
   d. subpoena duces tecum

3. Publicizing a patient's pregnancy would be:
   a. negligence
   b. invasion of privacy
   c. malpractice
   d. tort

4. When the patient makes an appointment with the doctor and shows up for that appointment, the doctor and patient have a/an:
   a. contract
   b. arbitration
   c. privileged communication
   d. tort

5. LSD belongs in which schedule of controlled drugs?
   a. I
   b. II
   c. III
   d. IV
   e. V

6. The schedule that includes drugs with the least potential for abuse is:
   a. I
   b. II

c. III
d. IV
e. V

7. The Truth-in-Lending Act states that any medical bill paid in ___ installments must show whether or not interest will be charged.
   a. more than three
   b. more than four
   c. two
   d. more than two

8. Malpractice can be avoided by:
   a. performing beyond your scope of practice
   b. keeping patients' complaints from the doctor
   c. practicing sepsis
   d. documenting all pertinent patient information

9. Informed consent is legal when:
   a. the patient signs a paper
   b. the patient knows all possible risks of a procedure
   c. the patient is told by the medical assistant about the surgery
   d. the patient is coerced into signing the consent

10. A living will is legal when:
    a. a doctor signs for the patient
    b. one witness is present when the patient signs
    c. the competent patient signs
    d. a patient on high doses of morphine signs

Answers

1. **d** Physicians are required to report vital statistics, communicable diseases, known or suspected abuse, drug abuse, and criminal acts.

2. **c** "Let the master answer" is the same as the doctrine of respondeat superior. It means that the doctor is responsible for the acts of the medical assistant.

3. **b** Publicizing a patient's pregnancy is invasion of privacy.

4. **a** When the patient makes an appointment with the doctor and shows up for that appointment, the doctor and the patient have a contract.

5. **a** LSD belongs to Schedule I drugs, the category that is not legalized and has the highest potential for abuse.

6. **e** The schedule of drugs with the least potential for abuse is Schedule V.

7. **b** The federal Truth-in-Lending Act states that any medical bill paid in more than four installments must show whether or not interest will be charged.

8. **d** Malpractice can be avoided by documenting all pertinent patient information.

9. **b** Informed consent is legal when the patient has been told all possible risks of a procedure.

10. **c** A living will can be valid only if the patient is competent at the time of signature and two witnesses are present.

6

Written Communication

CHAPTER OUTLINE

Formats
Editing

I. FORMATS

Standard stationery in a professional medical office is usually 16- to 24-pound weight and 8 ½ by 11 inches. Elite type is the best choice for professional correspondence.

   A. Letters

      1. *Full block:* date, inside address, salutation, body, complimentary closing, typed signature, and initials are flush left margin

         a. No tabs needed

Tony Moore, M.D.
100 Drivers Lane
Winterville, NC 28590

August 4, 1994

Jarrett Tucker, M.D.
Greenville Boulevard
Hills Point, NC 48567

Dear Doctor Tucker:

I appreciate your referring Jeff Stallings. He was seen in our office today. My examination revealed nothing remarkable.

I am requesting a CAT scan of the brain. His appointment is 8-16-94. He will return on 8-20-94 to discuss the scan.

Sincerely yours,

Tony Moore, M.D.

aph

Figure 6-1 Full block format.

2. _Modified block:_ date, complimentary closing, and typed signature a little to the right of center, with all three lining up
  a. Professional-looking with most letterheads

Tony Moore, M.D.
100 Drivers Lane
Winterville, NC 28590

August 4, 1994

Jarrett Tucker, M.D.
Greenville Boulevard
Hills Point, NC 48567

Dear Doctor Tucker:

Jeff Stallings

I appreciate your referring Jeff Stallings. He was seen in our office today. My examination revealed nothing remarkable.

I am requesting a CAT scan of the brain. His appointment is 8-16-94. He will return on 8-20-94 to discuss the scan.

Sincerely yours,

Tony Moore, M.D.

aph

Figure 6-2 Modified block format.

3. *Modified block with indented paragraphs:* date, complimentary closing, and typed signature a little to the right of center, all three lining up; each paragraph usually indented five spaces
   a. Least popular, probably because of the time it takes to tabulate

---

Tony Moore, M.D.
100 Drivers Lane
Winterville, NC 28590

August 4, 1994

Jarrett Tucker, M.D.
Greenville Boulevard
Hills Point, NC 48567

Dear Doctor Tucker:

I appreciate your referring Jeff Stallings. He was seen in our office today. My examination revealed nothing remarkable.

I am requesting a CAT scan of the brain. His appointment is 8-16-94. He will return on 8-20-94 to discuss the scan.

Sincerely yours,

Tony Moore, M.D.

aph

Figure 6-3 Modified block with indented paragraphs.

4. *General rules*
   a. *Months:* spelled out
   b. *Doctors:* use Joe Barnes, M.D. instead of Dr. Joe Barnes
   c. *Salutation:* followed by a colon in professional correspondence
   d. Double spacing between paragraphs
   e. First word only of the closing is capitalized (Yours truly)
   f. *Elite:* 12 characters per inch (usual professional type)
   g. *Pica:* 10 characters per inch (good for reports and speeches)
   h. Second pages
      • Name of addressee typed on seventh line
      • Page number
      • Date
      • Body of letter typed on tenth line

B. Memos

   1. Margin: flush left and double spaced; four lines of headings (names, date, and subject information) should line up on tabulation at tenth space as shown next:

MEMORANDUM

MEMO TO: Virginia Perkins, Manager

FROM: Jenny Hemby

DATE: January 9, 1994

SUBJECT: Annual Evaluations

(Leave two blank lines before the body of MEMORANDUM, and single-space body)

   2. No paragraph indention
   3. 2-inch top margin for a full sheet; 1-inch top margin for a half sheet

C. Reports

   1. Add ½ inch to the left margin (or margin and tab stops three spaces to the right), if bound
   2. Paragraphs indented five spaces
   3. Double space
   4. First page, 2-inch top margin; other pages, 1-inch top margin
   5. Bottom margin: 1 inch

D. Tables

   1. All-cap single-spaced title
   2. Body is centered horizontally
   3. Word columns align left; number columns align right
   4. Decimals aligned

E. Manuscripts

   1. Format is the same as that of bound reports

II. EDITING

A. *Watermark:* a mark seen through bond paper when held up to the light

   1. *Correct side of bonded paper:* type on paper in same direction as watermark can be read

B. *Erasable bond:* type on the correct side (erasable side)

C. Proofreader's Marks

∧	Insert comma	∨	Insert apostrophe
ᵛ ᵛ	Insert quotation marks	⊙	Insert period
⊙	Insert colon	;)	Insert semicolon
?/	Insert question mark	=/	Insert hyphen
ℓ	Delete	⊂	Close up
¶	Paragraph	∽	Transpose
⌗	Insert space	⊏	Move left
⊐	Move right	ꜱᴘ	Spell out
caps ≡	Capitals	/lc	Lower case

QUESTIONS

Choose the answer that will correct the underlined mistake, or leave as is if underlined portion has no mistake.

1.   November 3, 1993

Dr. James Barnes
1104 State Road
Winterville, NC 28590

   a. Dr. James Barnes, M.D.
   b. Doctor James Barnes
   c. James Barnes, M.D.
   d. leave as is

2. I appreciate your help very much.

                Yours Truly,

   a. Yours truely,
   b. Yours truly,
   c. Yours Truely,
   d. leave as is

3. Dear Mr. Perkins:
   a. Dear Mr. Perkins;
   b. Dear Mister Perkins;
   c. My dear Mr. Perkins,
   d. leave as is

4. Memo To: Gene Hemby
   From: James Langston

   a. MEMO TO: Gene Hemby
      FROM: James Langston
   b. MEMO TO: Gene Hemby
      FROM: James Langston
   c. Memo To: Gene Hemby
      From: James Langston
   d. leave as is

5. Move margins and tabs of bound reports three spaces to the right.
   a. five spaces right
   b. five spaces left
   c. three spaces left
   d. leave as is

Answers

1.   c   "James Barnes, M.D." is the correct way to write a physician's name in the inside address.

2.   b   "Yours truly," is correctly written with the first letter of the first word of the complimentary closing in caps and the second word in lowercase letters and punctuated with a comma following.

3.   d   The salutation is correct as is and is correctly punctuated with a colon.

4.   a   A memo heading should be double spaced, lined up flush left margin, and the information following each line of the heading should be at space 10 for the tabulation.

5.   d   The sentence is correct as is. A bound report should have the margins and tabs moved three spaces to the right to make room for the binding.

7

Office
Equipment

CHAPTER OUTLINE

General Office Machines
Computers

I. GENERAL OFFICE MACHINES
  A. Calculator/adding machine
      1. *Features:* digital display and tape for permanent record
      2. *Use:* billing, bank deposits, daily reports, and financial trans-
         actions
  B. Copy machine
      1. *Features:* different-sized papers, contrast, and settings for
         number of copies, size reduction, and size increase
      2. *Use:* copying instruction sheets, correspondence for patient
         files, reports, and bills
  C. Check writer
      1. *Features:* settings for date, name of payee, and amount of
         check
      2. *Use:* for writing checks that cannot be altered
  D. Postage meter and scales
      1. *Features:* prints postage on the envelope or on tabs to put
         on the envelope
      2. *Use:* scales weigh mail to obtain accurate postages and
         meters dispense exact postage; letters do not have to be can-
         celed or postmarked (saving time)
  E. Intercom, voice mail, and electronic mail
      1. *Features:* can be part of a telephone system
          a. *Intercom:* can transfer calls or speak within the office
             without yelling
          b. *Voice mail:* recording gives prompts for person calling to
             touch certain numbers and then record a message
          c. *E-mail:* with recordings and prompts, can send a mes-
             sage to the electronic mailbox via a fax machine
      2. *Use:* for paging parties to the phone or speaking from one
         room to the next; interoffice oral communication
  F. Beeper
      1. *Features:* compact and mobile
      2. *Use:* can be worn anywhere, so office staff can be in touch
         with the person wearing the beeper at all times
  G. Fax (facsimile) machine
      1. *Features:* quick means of sending and receiving information
         on paper through use of telecommunications
      2. *Use:* can quickly send lab reports, physical findings, and so
         on, from one place to another via telecommunications
          a. Confidentiality must still be practiced with fax machines
  H. Dictation machines
      1. *Features:* speed up, slow down, replay, foot pedals, and ear-
         phones
      2. *Use:* listen to doctor's notes for transcribing

I. Answering machines

    1. *Features:* settings for number of rings before pickup, can record and change own message, call back for messages, replay, rewind, and fast forward

    2. *Use*

        a. Answers phone and records message of caller

        b. Screens incoming calls prior to answering

II. COMPUTERS

  A. Terminology

    1. *Disk drive:* unit in which a diskette is inserted to obtain information from or to put information onto a diskette

    2. *Screen or monitor:* unit that displays processed information

    3. *Function keys:* keys for performing certain tasks (as in centering) and help keys (help-key: usually F1 but can vary depending on the software package)

    4. *Backup:* copies of existing data are available so that information will not be lost

    5. *Cursor:* a marker that shows where the next character will be typed or the next function will take place

    6. *Fonts:* character types

    7. *Hard copy:* the printout on paper of information from the screen

    8. *Initialize or format:* prepare a diskette for information storage

    9. *Menu:* display of functions from which to choose

    10. *Peripheral:* anything added to or plugged into the computer

    11. *Software:* various programs that direct the computer to do certain functions

    12. *Scrolling:* moving up or down through information

    13. *Modem:* connects computer to other computers for communication via telephone lines

        a. Dictation to another computer by phone

        b. Electronic claims processing

        c. Voice mail

    14. *CPU:* central processing unit

    15. *Hardware:* physical equipment (CPU, printer, keyboard, and monitor)

    16. *Password:* any alphanumeric series used as a way to get into a secured menu (e.g., payroll)

    17. *Tutorial:* a program that teaches use of the software

    18. *Commands:* certain words and symbols in a form and sequence to get the computer to do certain tasks (e.g., the command "Format a:" will format a disk)

  B. Uses

    1. Word processing

        a. Patient data input

        b. Correspondence

    c. Reports

    d. Patient educational materials

2. Billing and financial transactions (can process superbills for each patient daily with procedures and diagnoses and their CPT, ICD-9 CM, and HCPCS codes)

3. Insurance processing

    a. Electronic claims processing by telecommunication

4. Payroll

5. Year-end reports

6. Aging accounts

7. Activity analysis

8. Appointment scheduling

9. Accounts receivable reports (total amount all patients owe)

10. End-of-month statements

11. Database of all patients

C. Maintenance

  1. Instruction booklets to be read and followed

  2. Maintenance contracts and service agreements for designated price per month or year

  3. Computer diskettes

    a. Disk varieties

      • Size of diskettes: 3.5, 5.25, and 8 inches

      • Density of diskettes: DD (double density), HD (high density), and SD (single density)

      • Types of diskettes: hard and floppy

    b. Maintenance

      • No temperature extremes

      • Avoidance of dust, smoke, food, drink, and magnetic fields

      • Any label must be written on before attaching to the diskette, or written with a soft-tip pen

      • Diskette must never be forced into the drive

Match lettered items with the correct numbered statements.

a. Calculator
b. Copy machine
c. Check writer
d. Postage meter
e. Postage scales
f. Intercom
g. Beeper
h. Fax machine

h 1. A quick means of sending written information using telecommunications

f 2. A means of communicating orally from room to room

c 3. Features settings for date, name of payee, and amounts

a 4. Used for financial transactions using numerical functions

g 5. Device that can be worn so that a message to call back may be transmitted

d 6. Dispenses exact postage to be printed on an envelope

e 7. Weighs mail for exact postage

b 8. When corresponding with a patient, use this machine to make a second letter to file in chart

a. Monitor
b. Backup
c. Cursor
d. Initialize
e. Software
f. Hard copy
g. Scroll
h. Modem

g 9. Moving up or down through information

a 10. Display of information appears on this

b 11. Will not lose information if these copies called _____ are made

h 12. Connection of computers via telephone lines

f 13. Printed information from the screen

c 14. Marker showing where the next function will take place or the next character will be written

e 15. Programs that direct the computer to do various functions

d 16. Preparing a diskette for storage of information

Answers

1. h Fax machines send written communication via telephone lines from a fax machine in one place to a fax machine in another place.
2. f Intercoms make it easy to speak to a person in another room.
3. c Check writers have settings for the date, the payee, and the amount of the check.
4. a Calculators enable a person to do simple arithmetic automatically.
5. g It is possible to call a number that will cause a beep and alert the person wearing the beeper to call a certain number.
6. d Postage meters dispense the exact amount of postage needed and print it on the envelope or on a tab to be put on the envelope.

7. e Postage scales are used for weighing mail in order to figure the correct amount of postage.
8. b Copy machines are used to make copies of patient instruction sheets and correspondence or copies of other information necessary in a physician's office.
9. g Scrolling is moving up or down through information on the computer monitor.
10. a Monitors or screens display information put into the computer.
11. b Backup must be done daily or more frequently to ensure that information put into a computer is saved periodically so as not to be lost. It involves making copies of computer information on another diskette or tape cartridge.

12. **h** Modems are connectors of computers for communication via telephone lines.

13. **f** Hard copies are any printouts of computer information from the screen onto paper.

14. **c** A cursor shines or blinks at the place where the next character will be typed or the next function will take place.

15. **e** Software packages direct the computer to do special functions especially covered by that particular package.

16. **d** To initialize or format a diskette is to make it ready for receiving information from the computer.

8

Medical
Records

CHAPTER OUTLINE

Maintenance
Storage and Equipment
Confidentiality
Format

I. MAINTENANCE

   A. Supplies

      1. *Tabs:* for color coding names, dates, insurance, and so on

      2. *Folders:* condition (repair) folders when necessary

      3. *Outguides and outfolders:* may tell where a chart is or give a place to put papers until the chart is replaced

   B. Shingling: placing reports one over the other with bottom tab showing for organization

   C. Filing systems

      1. *Geographic:* file by area or location

      2. *Chronologic:* file by date

         a. *Tickler file:* a reminder system set up like a calendar by dates

      3. *Alphabetic:* file by ABC order, usually last name (surname) first

         Example: Langston, Betty

         a. "Nothing before something"
         Example: Smith is filed before Smithson

         b. "Last the same, try first name"
         Example: Langston, Blake before Langston, Jim

         c. When THE is part of a business name, consider it the last indexing unit
         Example: The Dime Store: Unit 1 = Dime, Unit 2 = Store, Unit 3 = The

         d. Titles are not considered
         Example: Professor John Smith and Sam Smith Smith, John (Professor) first, then Smith, Sam

         e. Hyphenated names are considered one unit
         Example: Jones-Johnson, John before Jonesrude, John

      4. *Numeric:* file by a numbering system, usually the smallest number to the largest disregarding any zeros in front of a number
         Example: 0012 before 014

         a. Cross-reference needed to be able to look up a patient's name alphabetically to find their chart number

         b. Terminal digit: in numbers such as 22-33-45, use the last two digits to sort files first, then the middle digits, then the first digits
         Example: 22-33-45 before 22-35-45

      5. *Subject:* file by heading or subject area

         a. Subject list needed for ease in filing

   D. Filing steps

      1. *Inspection and release:* checking to see if all action on information is completed before filing
      Example: doctor looks at lab report and initials it before it can be filed

      2. *Indexing:* deciding under which subject the information should be filed

3. _Coding:_ marking to show under which subject the information is to be filed
4. _Sorting:_ organizing material to be filed before actually filing it
5. _Storing:_ locating the proper place for filing and storing the information

II. STORAGE AND EQUIPMENT

  A. _File cabinets:_ Vertical, lateral, drawer, automatic, and shelf

  B. _Card index files_

  C. _Microfilm and diskettes_

  D. _Inactive files:_ files of patients who have not been seen in a specified period of time or of patients who have died; may be stored in special boxes in controlled storage

III. CONFIDENTIALITY

  A. Files are not released without patient authorization

    1. Release of records form must be signed by the patient

  B. Numerical filing is more confidential than alphabetical filing because a cross-reference is required

  C. Electronic information sent by Fax or computer is treated with the same rules of confidentiality

IV. FORMAT

  A. POMR: problem oriented medical record

    1. Organization by patient's problems instead of traditional source-oriented record (information sorted according to who generates it, such as nurses' notes, doctors' notes, or medical assistants' notes)

    2. _Database:_ patient information

    3. _Problems:_ any problems needing management will be in SOAP notes or progress notes form; always dated

      a. S = subjective: what patient tells office staff
      Example: "My foot hurts"

      b. O = objective findings: what health care worker (doctor, medical assistant, etc.) finds upon examination
      Example: v/s = T 101 P 72 R 14 B/P 120/90, x-ray-normal

      c. A = assessment: same as Dx (diagnosis)
      Example: A: Arthritis
      Example: A: R/O Arthritis
      Example: A: Arthritis vs. Bursitis

      d. P = plan
      Example: P: ii Getwell tabs TID, Re-check 1 wk.
      Example: P: Chest x-ray, PA and Lat STAT, F/U 1 week

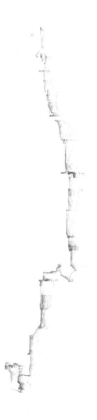

B. Corrections

    1. No erasing or whiting out; chart is written in black ink, so mark through once, initial, date, and make corrections above or beside. Some may choose to also write "corr" beside errors.

QUESTIONS

1. Explain the use of outguides or outfolders.
2. Define conditioning with regard to file management.
3. Name and define five filing systems.
4. Arrange the following in proper sequence from first to last:

a. Smith, Jane   b. Candy Store

Smith-Langston, Janet   The Best Candy Store

Langston, Betty

Smithson, Robert   c. 22-34-67

Dr. James Langston   23-33-66

5. Describe the format for progress notes under the POMR system.
6. Write the letter S, if subjective; the letter O, if objective; the letter A, if assessment; and the letter P, if plan.

   A a. Carpal tunnel syndrome
   O b. OU-PERRLA
   S c. "My throat hurts"
   A d. Fracture of left femur
   P e. Fleets enema x 3
   S f. "I have been coughing for three days"

Answers

1. Outguides are placed in the space where the folder or chart would normally be filed. They save the space for the chart and make it easier to file the chart in its correct space. Outfolders perform the same function as outguides except that they include a compartment for storage of papers that will be filed in the chart when it is replaced.

2. Conditioning is the act of maintaining and repairing charts when they are torn or need tabs replaced.

3.
   1 Geographic: file by location or area
   2 Chronologic: file by time or dates, such as the tickler file—like a calendar with reminder notes on each date.
   3 Subject: file by subject headings.
   4 Alphabetic: file by ABC sequence, names are usually alphabetized by last name, then first name, then middle initial.
   5 Numeric: file charts according to numerical order and according to type of system used (sequential terminal digit, etc.).

4. a Langston, Betty (Alphabetically, B comes before J, last name same, try first name.)
   Langston, James (L comes before S in Smith.)
   Smith, Jane (Nothing comes before something, nothing after Smith; Langston is presumed part of the name Smith-Langston.)
   Smith-Langston, Janet
   Smithson, Robert (Smith-Langston is treated as one name, so L comes before S in Smithson.)

   b The Best Candy Store comes before Candy Store. THE is considered the last indexing unit. Then, comparing BEST to CANDY, B comes before C in the alphabet.

   c In sequential filing, 22-34-67 comes before 23-33-66; however, the same numbers filed by the terminal digit method would be filed as 23-33-66, then 22-34-67, because the last two digits are the digits to be arranged sequentially in terminal-digit filing.

5. The format for progress notes using the POMR (problem oriented medical record) system is SOAP: S = subjective findings, O = objective findings, A = assessment or diagnosis, P = plan of action.

6. a A = assessment: carpal tunnel syndrome is a diagnosis.

   b O = objective findings by the health care worker: when shining a penlight in the eyes (OU), it is found that pupils are equal, round, and reactive to light and accommodation (PERRLA).

   c S = subjective: "My throat hurts" is something the patient says about himself/herself.

   d A = assessment: fracture of left femur is a diagnosis.

   e P = plan: Fleets enema x 3 is the doctor's plan for the patient to have three Fleet enemas.

   f S = subjective: "I have been coughing for three days" is something the patient says about himself/herself.

9

Postal Services

CHAPTER OUTLINE

Classes
Formats

I. CLASSES (BASED ON TYPE, WEIGHT AND DESTINATION)

   A. First class: 12 oz or less

      1. Letters and postcards, sealed or not sealed

      2. Green-diamond bordered envelopes

      3. Not subject to inspection

   B. Second class

      1. Newspapers and magazines

      2. Bulk mail sent by publishers and others

   C. Third class: up to 16 oz

      1. Catalogs and photographs

      2. Subject to inspection

   D. Fourth Class: 16 oz or more up to 70 lb (parcel post); maximum dimensions—108 inches, combined length and width

      1. Books, films, and manuscripts

   E. Combination mailing

      1. *Letter and package:* if a letter is inside a package, separate postage must be paid for each, and "letter enclosed" must be written on the package

   F. Educational materials

      1. Lower rate than fourth class

   G. Special services

      1. *Special delivery:* same speed of service from city to city, but will be delivered immediately upon arrival to the place of address if served by carriers or within 1 mile of the post office

      2. *Express mail:* high-speed delivery; sent by 5 P.M. one day and received by 3 P.M. the next day if delivered, but received by 10 A.M. if picked up by the receiver

      3. *Certificate of mailing:* receipt is evidence that item was mailed

      4. *Certified mail:* first-class mail with proof of delivery on record for 2 years

      5. *Registered mail:* evidence of delivery and added protection; person receiving must sign for mail; any class can be registered; especially useful for items of high value

      6. *Insured mail:* third and fourth class should be insured if the value is over $25

      7. *Receipt of delivery:* shows date item was received by the person to whom it was sent

      8. *Money orders:* safe way of sending money through the mail

      9. *Recall of mail:* written request with proper ID, mailer pays expenses

     10. *Priority mail:* exceptions to limitations of classes may be sent by "priority" to receive expeditious handling

        a. Rates based on weight and distance

11. *Address correction requested:* used to locate someone who has moved
    a. Post office will forward mail with "address correction requested" and send mailer new address for a fee

H. Alternatives to postal service

    1. Private services, such as UPS and Federal Express

    2. Couriers hired by private concerns, such as laboratories that pick up lab specimens

II. FORMATS

A. OCR read area

    1. Automation requires address within a rectangle that is 1 inch from right and left edges, $\frac{5}{8}$ inch and $2\text{-}\frac{3}{4}$ inches up from the bottom

    2. USPS bar code sprayed in the bottom right edge for further processing after OCR (optical character reader) reads address

B. Sans-serif characters best; script, handwriting, and italics cannot be read by the OCR

C. Maximum contrast best

D. Correct spacing between letters

E. All caps and no punctuation

F. Standard USPS state abbreviations

G. ZIP code on same line as city and state

    1. ZIP code should be 5+4 digits

    2. Nothing below ZIP code line

QUESTIONS

Match lettered items with the correct numbered items.

 a. First class
 b. Second class
 c. Third class
 d. Fourth class
 e. Educational materials
 f. Special delivery
 g. Certificate of mailing
 h. Receipt of delivery
 i. Registered mail

_e_ 1. Films mailed to a school

_c_ 2. Catalogs weighing up to 16 oz

_a_ 3. Letters and postcards

_i_ 4. Extra protection and proof of delivery for any class of mail

_g_ 5. Shows evidence that the item was mailed

_f_ 6. Delivery same from city to city but delivered immediately to destination upon arrival at post office

_h_ 7. Gives proof that the item was delivered

_b_ 8. Newspapers and magazines

_d_ 9. Parcel post

10. Explain how to address an envelope for automated delivery.

Answers

1. e   A film mailed to a school is mailed at a lower rate than fourth class and classified as educational material.

2. c   Catalogs weighing up to 16 oz are considered third class mail.

3. a   Letters and postcards are considered first-class mail.

4. i   Registered mail gives further protection and proof of delivery for any class of mail.

5. g   Certificate of mailing shows evidence of mailing.

6. f   Special delivery speeds up delivery after the item has reached the designated post office. After arrival, the item is delivered immediately to its destination.

7. h   Receipt of delivery gives proof that the item reached its destination.

8. b   Second-class postage is the classification used for newspapers and magazines.

9. d   Fourth class is considered parcel post. Packages may weigh 16 oz or more, but cannot weigh over 70 lb.

10.   For automation, an address must be within the boundaries of an imaginary rectangle that is $5/8$ inch and $2\text{-}3/4$ inches from the bottom, with right and left margins of 1 inch. The letters are best read if they are sans serif, have maximum contrast, are all capitalized, without punctuation, are spaced well, and have the ZIP code on the same line as the city and the standard state abbreviation.

10

Appointment Processes

CHAPTER OUTLINE

Schedules
Guidelines

I. SCHEDULES

   A. *Open office hours:* no appointment necessary; patients can come in at any time the office is open

      1. Most common appointment system for emergency medical centers

   B. *Time-specified appointments:* each patient is given a certain time to arrive

   C. *Wave scheduling:* more than one patient is given a time on the hour to come, but then patients are seen on a first come, first served basis. Duration of patients' total appointments is equal to or less than an hour.

      1. Allowance for early and late arrivals

      2. Attempt to start and finish each hour on time

   D. *Double booking:* two people given the same appointment time

      1. Not a good practice; duration of the patients' total appointment time is more than the time available on appointment book

   E. Patient's total waiting time should be no more than 20 minutes

      1. Sign-in sheet made available with times checked by staff frequently

      2. Sign should be posted at the front desk requesting patient to alert staff if the wait is more than 20 minutes or other specified time

   F. Blank spaces should be left in the schedule for work-ins, emergencies, and so on

      1. Work-ins usually handled before lunch and in the late afternoon

      2. If there are no work-ins, the time is used to catch up on the schedule

   G. *Categorizing appointments:* doctors may wish to see all surgery patients on one day or all routine physicals on one afternoon

II. GUIDELINES

   A. Familiarization with types of appointments, treatments and their duration, and doctors' individual habits is necessary to schedule effectively

   B. Familiarization with facilities, specialty examination rooms, and equipment is needed

   C. Matrix (cross out times for vacations, surgery, meetings, lunch, etc.) must be established before making appointments

   D. Missed and canceled appointments should be noted on the patient's chart with the reason

   E. Attempts to reschedule missed and cancelled appointments should be made with notation on the chart that rescheduling attempts were made

   F. *Information necessary to write down for each appointment:* name, phone number, and chief complaint

G. *Miscellaneous information needed:* whether established or new patient, whether referred and by whom, date of birth, chart number, and address

H. *Doctor delays:* always explain to the patient and give them a choice to reschedule or wait

I. *Emergencies:* must triage and see according to severity

J. *Patient need vs. preference for appointment time:* it is best to schedule for the patient's convenience unless another time is better (e.g., equipment needed for the patient will be in use; a diabetic patient should be seen soon after eating unless scheduled for specific tests)

K. *Cancellation list:* keep on hand so that schedule can be filled

L. *Doctor referrals:* to be seen as soon as possible

M. Keep list on hand for priority appointments

Decide in which category of appointment scheduling the following appointments belong: wave scheduling, double booking, time specified, or categorizing.

1. 8:00 Donna Corey-abdominal cramping (30 min.)

   Susan Moore—routine physical (30 min.)

   Jill Whichard—Follow-up sinusitis (15 min.)

2. 8:00 John Corey—headaches (15 min.)

   Jenny Hemby—routine physical (30 min.)

   Buddy Waters—otitis (15 min.)

3. 8:00 Chad Corey—nausea (15 min.)

   8:15 Christine Walters-routine physical (30 min.)

   8:30 ———————

   8:45 Chris West—fractured great toe (30 min.)

Fill in the blanks:

4. Before scheduling any appointment, one must first cross out times for surgery, meetings, and so on. This action is called _____ _____ _____.

5. A patient should never wait any longer than _twenty_ _minutes_.

6. The best times to leave spaces for catching up on the day's schedule are _before lunch_ and _late evening_

7. The three most important pieces of information to include about patients in their appointment slots are
   name,
   Phone, and
   _C/o_.

8. Open office hours are generally used by _walk in_ _Patient_.

Answers

1. Scheduling two 30-minute appointments and one 15-minute appointment within a time block of 1 hour would be considered double booking. The medical assistant has not allowed an adequate amount of time for the three appointments.

2. Assigning three or four appointments within an hour with the total time for all appointments in that hour not exceeding an hour is considered wave scheduling. Each hour patients will be scheduled as stated, and each hour should start and end on time. Wave scheduling attempts to start and end each hour on time.

3. A specific time indicated within each hour for each appointment is considered a time-specified appointment. Each person arrives at the appropriate time and should be seen as soon as possible thereafter.

4. Crossing out times for surgery, meetings, hospital rounds, and so on, on the appointment book is called establishing the matrix. After doing this, the medical assistant will know in what blocks of time patients can be scheduled for appointments with the doctor.

5. Good office management dictates that a patient should never wait more than 20 minutes. If a patient waits any longer than 20 minutes, the receptionist should acknowledge the fact, offer an explanation, and give the patient a choice of rescheduling.

6. Catching up time is usually needed before lunch and in the late afternoon. If blanks can be left in the schedule in those places, then any work-ins due to emergencies or acute illnesses can be seen by the doctor each day without putting her/him too far behind schedule.

7. The three most important pieces of information to include in the patients' appointment slots are the patient's name, chief complaint, and telephone number. The name, of course, has to be known. The chief complaint has to be known in order to know approximately how much time needs to be given to that appointment, and the telephone number is necessary in case the doctor has an emergency and the appointment has to be canceled. Other pieces of information sometimes elicited while scheduling appointments are whether or not the patient has been seen there before, if another doctor has referred the patient, the patient's date of birth, and the patient's chart number, if one has been assigned. Whether or not this information is included may be governed by the amount of space in the appointment book or the appointment scheduling software package.

8. Open office hours are usually used by emergency medical centers. Because of the nature of the complaint, and the fact that it is acute or an emergency, a patient could not generally make an appointment anyway.

11

Community Services

A medical assistant should be a patient advocate not only between the doctor and patient, but also between the patient and community resources. Knowledge of community resources will ultimately help all patients when their needs can be met by referral to community resources.

CHAPTER OUTLINE

Resources

I. RESOURCES
   A. *Hospitals*
      1. *General hospitals:* short-term hospitalization
      2. *Specialty hospitals:* hospitalization for specific diseases such as cancer and tuberculosis, or for psychiatric care
   B. *Surgical centers:* usually for outpatient surgeries
   C. *Emergency medical centers:* smaller than hospital emergency areas, usually for minor trauma
   D. *Convalescent care:* nursing homes, usually for long-term geriatric (elderly) care
   E. *Clinics:* various specialties in one office complex
   F. *Home health care agencies:* for patient care in the home
   G. *Senior day care:* elderly sitting services
   H. *Health department:* preventive health care, promotion of disease control, and public health education
   I. *Social services department:* financial aid and human resource aid, (e.g., Medicaid, food stamps, adult protection, child protection)
   J. *Volunteer agencies and support groups:* medical assistants should be familiar with their own community resources for referrals when needed for financial, emotional, or other kinds of support
      1. *American Cancer Society:* education, health fair participation, and cancer prevention
      2. *American Red Cross:* blood drives and emergency services
      3. *American Heart Association:* wellness education and prevention of heart disease
      4. *American Diabetes Association:* diabetes education
      5. *Hospice:* for dying patients and their families
      6. *Council on Aging:* home-delivered meals, legal and insurance information, help for neglected seniors, and transportation assistance
      7. *Lions Club:* financial support for the visually impaired
      8. *Children's services:* help for cases of abuse or neglect and financial assistance
      9. *Handicapped and developmental services:* evaluation, management, and rehabilitation
      10. *Drug and alcohol abuse services:* education and rehabilitation
      11. *Rehabilitation services:* mental, physical, and drug abuse, and cases with vocational and counseling services
      12. *American Lung Association:* education, smoking cessation clinics, and support groups
      13. *Weight control and dietary services:* nutrition education and support groups

QUESTIONS

1. Name an agency responsible for educating the public about health maintenance.

2. Name an agency or support group that might financially assist a visually impaired patient.

3. Families requesting care for a patient in the home would contact what agency?

4. Name five support groups in your community.

Answers

1. Your county health department endeavors to educate the public about communicable diseases, holistic health, maternal and child care, disease prevention, and health maintenance, among other things.

2. The Lion's Club may assist a visually impaired patient financially.

3. A home health care agency may place a health care worker in the home to provide health care service.

4. Answers may vary.

12

Office Management

CHAPTER OUTLINE

Editorial and Travel Duties
Policies and Procedures/Office Management
Accounting/Financial Management
Inventory
Physical Plant
Liability Coverage

I. EDITORIAL AND TRAVEL DUTIES
  A. Office library
    1. Physician's journals
      a. *JAMA (Journal of the American Medical Association)*
      b. Specialty journals
    2. Patient educational materials
      a. Videos
      b. Disease brochures
      c. Models
    3. Organization
      a. *Card catalog:* author, title, and subject
      b. Abstracts may summarize and file the most important points of an article
      c. Journals bound and index of contents made
  B. Research
    1. Materials search
      a. Card catalog
      b. Periodical index *(Index Medicus)*
      c. Computer search
      d. Bibliography list
  C. Speech typing
    1. Double space
  D. *Arrangement of meetings:* block out meetings on the appointment schedule and reschedule appointments if necessary or assign coverage for those attending the meetings.
    1. Reason for meeting
    2. Place
    3. Time
    4. Date
    5. Duration
    6. Expected attendance
    7. Announcement of meeting
    8. Food requirements (refreshments or meals)
    9. *Agenda:* items to be discussed at the meeting
    10. Minute taking
      a. Presider
      b. Name of association
      c. Date, time, place, and type of meeting
      d. Those present
      e. Minutes read and approved
      f. Items of business, and any motions made and by whom made
      g. Hour of adjournment

E. *Travel arrangements:* block out times for travel on the appointment schedule and assign coverage or reschedule appointments.
   1. Preparation of itinerary
   2. Motel reservations, confirmation of reservations, and late arrival guarantee
   3. Method of transportation
   4. Date and time of departure and return
   5. Purchase of necessary tickets
   6. Mailing of necessary registration
   7. Inclusion of maps, brochures, other necessary information
F. Patient instruction and information booklets
   1. Booklets updated and sent to patients to introduce them to the practice or to acquaint them with their diseases

II. POLICIES AND PROCEDURES/OFFICE MANAGEMENT
   A. Policy manual/personnel
      1. Philosophy of the office
      2. Line-of-authority chart
      3. Policies of the office
         a. *Interviewing, hiring, and firing*
            • Knowledge of fair employment practice laws is necessary
            • Same questions should be asked of each interviewee so that a fair evaluation can be made
            • All applicants should be notified when positions are filled
            • Exit interviews should be conducted when employees leave
            • Warnings and documentation should be provided during evaluations so that the employees may have a chance to improve unless circumstances (e.g., stealing, insubordination) require immediate dismissal
         b. *Sick leave and vacation:* established policies are necessary for all employees
         c. *Evaluation of personnel*
            • Probationary period: a specific period of time before the employee is hired permanently
            • Documentation of all evaluations
            • Regular reviews
         d. *Dress code:* should be established and adhered to
         e. *Other office management*
            • Staff meetings when necessary
            • Harmony of staff included in management
            • Work flow/patient flow: manager monitors equality of workload and flow of patients and makes changes when necessary
      4. *Office maintenance:* equipment justification, ordering, and maintenance, and housekeeping

B. Procedure manual
   1. *Job descriptions:* can consult *DOT (Dictionary of Occupational Titles)*
   2. Step-by-step guide for carrying out each job in the office
   3. Guide for the clinical setups (minor surgery setups, specialty procedures, and so on)

III. ACCOUNTING/FINANCIAL MANAGEMENT
   A. Payroll
      1. Employee information
         a. Name
         b. Social Security number
         c. Exemptions and deductions
         d. Gross salary (before taxes) or hourly wage
         e. Amount of overtime if applicable
         f. Marital status and length of pay period (for income tax withheld)
      2. Forms
         a. *W-4 form:* withholding allowance certificate; shows the number of exemptions claimed
         b. *W-2 form:* wage and tax statement; given at the end of the year or by January 31 at the latest
         c. *Form 941:* employer's quarterly federal tax return
         d. *Form 940:* employer's annual federal unemployment tax return (FUTA)
      3. Taxes
         a. *FICA:* Federal Insurance Contributions Act
            • *OASI:* Old Age and Survivors Insurance
            • *HI:* hospitalization under Medicare
            • *DI:* disability insurance
         b. *FUTA:* Federal Unemployment Tax Act
         c. *FWT:* Federal withholding tax
         d. *SWT:* State withholding tax
         e. Local taxes in some areas
   B. Bank reconciliation
      1. Monthly bank statement
      2. Reconciliation of bank statement with checkbook balance
      3. Subtract bank fees (service charges, etc.) from checkbook balance and circle this figure as reconciliation 1
      4. Subtract outstanding checks from bank statement balance and add outstanding deposits to bank statement balance. Circle this figure as reconciliation 2
      5. Reconciliations 1 and 2 should be the same
   C. Check writing
      1. Stub of each check should have amount, date, payee, and purpose of the check
      2. Stub is filled out before removing the check

3. Check is voided if a mistake has been made
4. Acceptance of checks
    a. All spaces filled out correctly
    b. Third-party checks accepted only for payments by insurance companies
    c. Checks accepted only for the amount due
    d. Acceptance of no check marked "payment in full" unless it is, in fact, full payment
    e. *Endorsement:* on the back of check write "for deposit only" to ensure that the check can only be deposited into the proper account
D. Deposits to account
    1. Currency (paper money) listed first; face side up with larger bills on top and like denominations together
    2. Coin amount listed
    3. Checks recorded individually by ABA number (the fraction in the right upper corner) and amount of check
    4. Money orders and other types of payments recorded last
E. Accounts payable
    1. Bills paid by the physician's office are usually paid by check
    2. *Invoice (not a bill):* shows amount due and describes item
    3. *Statement:* bill for goods and materials received
    4. *Petty cash:* small amount of cash to have on hand for expenses and bills too small to require checks; instead one check is written "To Petty Cash" and the money put in a cash drawer to pay small bills
F. Accounts receivable
    1. *Amounts patients owe the physician:* best kept to minimum by collecting on day of service
    2. *Extending credit:* if amount to be paid is in more than four installments, a truth-in-lending statement must be signed (states whether or not interest will be charged)
    3. *Credit cards:* frequently accepted in the doctor's office for payments on a bill
    4. *Insurance payments:* patient must sign a record release form (patient is giving consent for the insurance company to know confidential information so that payment can be authorized) and Assignment of Benefits Form (so that payment will be made directly to the physician)
    5. *Cycle billing:* sending bills at different times of the month for smooth cash flow
    Example: send A to E on the first of the month; send F to J on the sixth; and send K to O on the twelfth
    6. *Delinquent accounts:* 120 days overdue or according to office policy; may be turned over to a collection agency
        a. Collection letters may be sent, and telephone calls made without harassment
        b. Requests for payment usually at 30, 60, and 90 days overdue

       c. Accounts sent to collection agency are flagged so that no more bills will be sent to the patient by the office

   7. *Collection ratio:* total payments YTD (year to date) divided by charges YTD, less adjustments; should be approximately 95 percent

   8. *Accounts receivable ratio:* accounts receivable balance divided by average gross monthly charges equals the average number of months in which accounts are being paid; should be less than two months

       a. Aging of accounts should be done monthly to increase collections efforts

   9. *Pegboard system:* "write it once"

       a. Superbill (charge slip, encounter form, receipt), ledger card, and journal (daysheet entry) all done at one time

       b. "Write it once" due to use of pegboard, shingled forms, ledger cards, and carbon transfers

       c. Computerized office equipment now replacing pegboard systems

IV. INVENTORY

   A. *Yearly:* for tax and depreciation purposes

   B. *Daily:* for ordering supplies as needed

   C. *Budget:* duty of management to evaluate needed equipment, justify need, and budget accordingly

V. PHYSICAL PLANT

   A. Maintenance of equipment, repairs of physical plant, safety of office, and so on, are all part of management

VI. LIABILITY COVERAGE

   A. Coverage for doctors and employees is a necessity

   B. Policies kept indefinitely

QUESTIONS

1. What three cards should be included in the card catalog for the medical office library?
2. _____ are summaries of important points in an article.
3. For easier delivery, speeches should be typed by _____ spacing.
4. List nine items that must be known prior to arranging a meeting.
5. List seven items to include when taking minutes of a meeting.
6. List seven items necessary for planning travel arrangements.
7. Explain the need for a policy manual and a procedure manual in a physician's office.
8. List two types of taxes withheld from an employee's paycheck.
9. What is a W-2 form?
10. What is a W-4 form?
11. Explain cycle billing.
12. What is the purpose of a federal truth-in-lending statement?
13. Explain a record release form pertaining to insurance billing.
14. Explain an assignment of benefits form.
15. Explain the method of listing money for a bank deposit.
16. Why does a medical office use petty cash?
17. Define accounts payable.
18. Define accounts receivable.
19. Reconcile the following bank statement and checkbook balance:

    Bank Statement=$700.00
    Checkbook balance=$895.00
    Bank fees=$5.00

    Outstanding check=$10.00
    Outstanding deposits= $100.00 and $100.00

Answers

1. An office library should have a title card, subject card, and author card for each item in the library.
2. Abstracts are summaries of important points in an article.
3. Speeches should be typed double spaced, for easiest reading and delivery.
4. When arranging a meeting, one needs to know the reason for the meeting, the time, the date, the place, how long the meeting will last, the number expected to attend, the method of announcing the meeting, the food requirements, (if any), and the agenda.
5. Minutes of a meeting should include who presided, name of association, date, time, and place of meeting, those present, approval of minutes, business items and motions made, and hour of adjournment.
6. Travel arrangements should include an itinerary, motel reservations, confirmations and late arrival guarantees, method of transportation, date and time of departure and return, ticket purchase, registration mailing, maps, and miscellaneous information.
7. Policy manuals explain the office philosophy, line of authority, and office regulations concerning sick leave, vacation, dress code, and so on. Procedure manuals are "how to" guides explaining step-by-step methods of office and clinical procedures.
8. The two taxes withheld from an employee's paycheck are FICA (Federal Insurance Contributions Act including hospitalization/Medicare, disability, and Old Age and Survivors Insurance) and FWT (federal withholding tax). State and local taxes may be withheld, depending on the area. FUTA (federal unemployment) is paid by the employer.
9. The W-2 form is given at the end of the year to show the total amount paid the employee during the year. It is called the wage and tax statement.
10. The W-4 form is filled out by the employee when hired. It shows the number of exemptions claimed by the employee so that the payroll clerk can figure the net pay. It is called the withholding allowance certificate.

11.   Cycle billing is done to ensure a smooth cash flow throughout the month. Instead of billing all patients at one time during the month, cycle billing provides for billing at spaced time intervals throughout the month.

12.   The federal truth-in-lending form is sent to any person paying in more than four installments. It includes a statement declaring whether or not interest is being charged.

13.   A record release form is signed by the patient to give permission to the physician's office to release to the insurance company information about the patient regarding diagnosis and other details so that the claim can be filed and paid.

14.   An assignment of benefits form is signed by the patient giving permission for the insurance company to pay the physician directly for the bill.

15.   Deposits are made by listing the paper money or currency first, coin amount next, checks individually itemized next, and money orders last. Currency should be organized with all money portrait side up, facing the same way.

16.   Petty cash is a small amount of cash on hand to pay small bills such as parking tickets.

17.   Accounts payable are bills to be paid by the doctor's office for items bought on credit.

18.   Accounts receivable are amounts that patients owe the doctor's office.

19.   Checkbook balance is $895.00. Bank fees are $5.00. The bank statement is $700.00. There are two outstanding deposits of $100.00 each. There is one outstanding check of $10.00.

Step one:
Checkbook balance - bank fees:
$895.00 - $5.00 = $890.00

Step two:
Add outstanding deposits to bank statement balance:
$200.00 + $700.00 = $900.00

Subtract outstanding checks:
$900.00 - $10.00 = $890.00
$890.00 = $890.00

13

Health Insurance

CHAPTER OUTLINE

Insurance Terminology
Types of Insurance
Filing of Claims

I. INSURANCE TERMINOLOGY

   A. _Assignment of benefits:_ specification of whom is to receive payment; if the patient signs a form assigning benefits to the doctor, the payment from the insurance company will be sent to the doctor

   B. _Deductible:_ predetermined amount to be paid "out of pocket" by the patient before insurance will begin to pay. If the deductible is $75.00, the patient must pay the first $75.00 of the bill; then the insurance will begin to pay its percentage

   C. _Co-payment:_ a designated amount or rate the patient must pay toward the bill; after the deductible has been met, the patient may have a $10.00 co-payment on each service thereafter or may pay a certain percentage of the bill

   D. _Fee schedule:_ a list of the fees charged for each service

   E. _Usual fee:_ the most prevalent fee doctors charge for each procedure

   F. _Customary fees:_ a range of fees that many doctors in a locale charge for each procedure

   G. _Reasonable fees:_ fees charged a patient when circumstances make the usual procedure more complicated

   H. _Precertification:_ prior authorization by an insurance company for payment for a specified procedure in the hospital

   I. _DRG (diagnostic related groups):_ for payment purposes, puts related diagnoses into groups according to procedures performed, patient's age, sex, discharge status, and complications/comorbidities

   J. _Coordination of benefits:_ if a patient is insured by more than one insurance company, the primary insurance company will pay first, the secondary insurance company will pay on the amount left, and so on; however, the total of all payments should be no more than 100 percent of the charges

II. TYPES OF INSURANCE

   A. _Medicaid:_ provides health care for the indigent

      1. Cards may be issued monthly so cards should be checked for current date (varies from state to state)

   B. _Medicare:_ two parts

      1. _Hospital (Part A):_ those receiving Social Security benefits automatically receive hospital benefits under Medicare

      2. _Medical (Part B):_ If a person receives Part A, she/he is eligible (there are others that may be eligible as well), but all must pay the premium monthly

   C. _CHAMPUS:_ Civilian Health and Medical Program of the Uniformed Services

   D. _CHAMPVA:_ Civilian Health and Medical Program of the Veterans Administration

E. *Blue Cross and Blue Shield:* medical and surgical insurance

    1. *Blue Cross:* hospitalization

    2. *Blue Shield:* physician's payments

F. *Workers' compensation:* covers the patient for loss of wages and provides health care when illness or injury is job related

    1. Doctor must file "Doctor's First Report of Occupational Injury" within 72 hours of the patient's first visit

III. FILING OF CLAIMS

A. Universal Claim Form: HCFA-1500

    1. First form completed without charge

    2. *Multiple forms:* justifiable for physician's office to charge for completion

    3. *Authorization to release information:* must be signed to give the office permission to release patient's confidential information

    4. *Assignment of benefits:* must be signed for payment to be sent directly to the provider

    5. Diagnostic codes must be correct and agree with procedure codes, and vice versa

    6. Dates should have six-digit format, 00/00/00

    7. Upgrading of knowledge of insurance codes and formats is a must for good reimbursement

B. Electronic claims filing

C. Rejections

    1. Diagnosis and treatment may not be relevant

    2. Incomplete forms

    3. Inaccurate coding

    4. Items incorrectly typed, such as date 10-1-93 not typed as 10-01-93

D. Coding

    1. ICD-9-CM: *International Classification of Diseases,* Ninth Revision, *Clinical Modification,* three volumes

        a. *Diseases:* tabular list

        b. *Diseases:* alphabetic index

        c. *Procedures:* tabular list and alphabetic index (not used in the physician's office)

        d. *Three-digit code that codes individual diseases:* add decimal and extra digits to code specificities about each disease.

    2. CPT-4: *Current Procedural Terminology,* five sections

        a. Medicine (evaluation and management codes located here)

        b. Anesthesiology

        c. Surgery

        d. Radiology

        e. Pathology and laboratory

     f. *Five-digit code that codes medical procedures:* add decimal and two digit modifier to show that a procedure has been altered

3. HCPCS: Health Care Financing Administration Common Procedure Coding System

     a. Five-digit Medicare alphanumeric codes based on CPT codes

     b. Three levels of coding

4. Superbills/encounter forms

     a. A listing of codes of possible services rendered

        • Diagnosis is entered, services rendered are circled, patient data is entered, and fees are entered

     b. *Completed superbill:* can sometimes be attached to the insurance form for filing the claim

Match the definition and the term.
   a. Coordination of benefits
   b. Assignment of benefits
   c. DRG
   d. Deductible
   e. Precertification
   f. Co-payment
   g. Fee schedule
   h. Usual fees
   i. Customary fees
   j. Reasonable fees

_g_ 1. A list of fees the insurance company will pay for each service

_j_ 2. Fees charged when circumstances make a procedure more complicated than normal

_h_ 3. Fees charged normally for each procedure

_g_ 4. A range of fees charged in a general locale

_a_ 5. No more than 100 percent of the bill will be paid by all insurance

_b_ 6. The payment of the bill will go directly to the physician if signed

_d_ 7. A predetermined amount a patient must pay before insurance will begin to pay

_c_ 8. Group related diagnoses according to procedure performed, patient's age, sex, and discharge status

_e_ 9. Prior authorization of payment for a hospital procedure

_f_ 10. After insurance begins to pay, the patient may have to pay a designated portion of each service

Match the type of insurance to the definition.
   a. Medicare
   b. Medicaid
   c. Blue Cross and Blue Shield
   d. CHAMPUS
   e. CHAMPVA
   f. Workers' compensation

___ 11. Reimburses for loss of wages due to job-related illness or accident

___ 12. Has Part A—Hospitalization and (if enrolled) Part B—Medical Insurance

___ 13. Insurance for dependents of those in the military and retirees and their dependents

___ 14. Insurance for spouses and dependent children of veterans

___ 15. Insurance for the medically indigent

___ 16. May provide medical, hospital, or surgical insurance for those who pay

Write the letter of the type of coding that matches the definition.
   a. CPT-4
   b. ICD-9-CM

___ 17. Uses a five-digit code (81000), decimal, then modifiers

___ 18. Uses a three-digit code (494), decimal, then modifiers

___ 19. Codes procedures

___ 20. Codes diseases or diagnoses

___ 21. Has tabular and alphabetic disease lists

___ 22. Has five sections

Answers

1. **g** A fee schedule lists amounts the insurance company will pay for services.

2. **j** Reasonable fees are charged when a procedure is more complicated than normal.

3. **h** Fees are termed "usual" when they are fees that the doctor normally charges for that procedure.

4. **i** Customary fees are a range of fees charged for procedures in a given area.

5. **a** Coordination of benefits is accomplished when no more than 100 percent of the bill is paid by the total of all insurance companies paying.

6. **b** Assignment of benefits forms are signed by the patient so that the payment for the bill will go directly to the doctor.

7. **d** A deductible is met when the patient pays a certain amount designated by the insurance company before the insurance company will pay any part of the bill.

8. **c** DRGs are diagnostic related groups that categorize a patient's hospital visit by procedure, patient's age, sex, discharge status, complications, and comorbidities.

9. **e** Precertification gives advance authorization for payment for a specified hospital procedure.

10. **f** Co-payments are a portion of a bill that is paid on each service after the deductible is met.

11. **f** Workers' compensation allows a worker to be reimbursed for wages lost due to a job-related illness or injury.

12. **a** Medicare has Part A—Hospitalization and Part-B—Medical.

13. **d** CHAMPUS is for those in the military and their dependents.

14. **e** CHAMPVA is for spouses and dependents of veterans.

15. **b** Medicaid is for the medically indigent or poor.

16. **c** BCBS, Blue Cross and Blue Shield, premiums may be paid for surgical, medical, and hospital insurance.

17. **a** CPT codes are five digits plus a decimal and modifier, if used.

18. **b** ICD-9-CM codes are three digits plus a decimal and modifier, if used.

19. **a** CPT codes procedures.

20. **b** ICD-9-CM codes diagnoses or diseases.

21. **b** ICD-9-CM has tabular and alphabetic disease lists.

22. **a** CPT has five sections: Medicine, Anesthesiology, Surgery, Radiology, and Pathology and Laboratory.

14

Infection Control

CHAPTER OUTLINE

Medical Asepsis
Surgical Asepsis

I. MEDICAL ASEPSIS

   A. *Clean technique* (as free of bacteria as possible): used during noninvasive procedures

      1. *Handwashing:* the single most important method of medical asepsis

         a. Wash hands thoroughly (may leave on gold band ring) with fingertips downward

      2. *Sanitization:* washing of items with detergent and water or antiseptic (used on living tissue)

      3. *Disinfection:* destroying many infectious organisms using chemicals (used on inanimate objects)

      4. Chain of transmission

         a. *Reservoir host:* provides nourishment for infection

         b. *Means of exit:* infectious organism exits through open wound or other body orifice

         c. *Transmission:* to another susceptible host through contact with a person or a person's infected waste or discharge (sneeze, feces) or contaminated objects

         d. *Means of entry:* infectious organism gains entry through the skin or a body orifice

      5. Breaking the chain

         a. Removal of nourishment necessary for infectious organism to live

            • Decrease oxygen if organism thrives on it

            • Change temperature if organism thrives at certain temperatures

            • Decrease moisture if organism thrives in a wet or moist environment

            • Increase light if organism thrives in darkness

      6. Universal blood and body fluid precautions

         a. *Barrier protection:* masks, gloves, gowns, aprons, and goggles

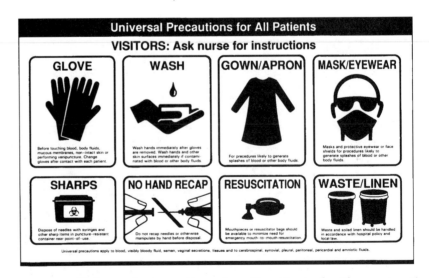

Figure 14-1   Universal precautions for all patients for the protection of patients, family, and health care workers.

B. Guarding against infectious agents
1. Bacteria: classified by morphology (size and shape)
   a. *Cocci:* round-shaped
   b. *Staphylococci:* round clusters of bacteria
   c. *Streptococci:* round bacteria in chains
   d. *Diplococci:* round bacteria in twos
   e. *Spirilla:* spiral-shaped bacteria
   f. *Bacilli:* rod-shaped bacteria
   g. *Chlamydia:* small bacteria that cannot live without a host
2. *Fungi:* yeasts and molds; vegetative organisms
3. *Rickettsiae:* parasites causing spotted fever and typhus
4. *Protozoa:* single-celled animals, usually nonparasitic
5. *Helminths:* parasitic worms
6. *Virus:* smaller than the microorganisms listed above
C. Medical examination instruments
1. *Otoscope:* for viewing the ear
2. *Ophthalmoscope:* for viewing the eye
3. *Stethoscope:* auscultation (listening) of heart, lungs, bowel sounds, and bruits (abnormal sounds); listening to the brachial artery during blood pressure checks
4. *Tuning fork:* checks sound perception (air and bone conduction)
5. *Reflex/percussion hammer:* checks reflexes (knee jerk, ankle jerk, brachioradialis, biceps, and triceps)
6. *Pinwheel:* checks sensations
7. *Laryngeal mirror:* views back of throat, tonsils, and adenoids
8. *Speculum:* opens area for viewing, inspection, examination, and passing instruments
   a. Vaginal
   b. Nasal
   c. Proctoscope
   d. Anoscope
9. *Lister bandage scissors:* cut through bandages; have blunt, rounded end

II. SURGICAL ASEPSIS
A. Guarding against infectious microorganisms during surgical or invasive techniques
1. *Sterilization:* complete destruction of all microorganisms, including spores
   a. *Autoclave* (e.g., pressurized steam at 15 pounds of pressure, 250° F, for 20 minutes): has variations of time, pressure, and temperature
   b. *Dry heat:* subject to high heat (165 to 170° C for 2 to 3 hours)

2. Sterile field setup and surgery
    a. *Skin prep:* swabbing skin, usually with a Betadine preparation to render it as free of pathogenic microorganisms as possible
    b. Sterile, nonfenestrated (no holes) drape over cleaned and dried tray or Mayo stand
    c. Fenestrated drape (has a hole in it so that the drape covers the surgical area but leaves an opening where the incision is to be made)
    d. All supplies, such as gauze sponges, sutures, needle holders, forceps, scissors, scalpels, cotton-tipped applicators, and cautery, must be sterile and "popped onto" or transferred to sterile field
        • Reaching over the sterile field = contamination
        • Anything below waist level is considered nonsterile
        • Anything touching outside a 1-inch border = contamination
        • Wetting of sterile field = contamination (unless it has a plastic barrier)
    e. Gloves, gown, masks, and any other barriers needed are set aside for donning by the doctor and assistants
        • Surgical scrub is necessary for the doctor and any assistants
        • Hands and arms are washed and scrubbed up to the elbows for a prescribed amount of time, fingernails are cleaned, and fingertips are held upward
        • No jewelry is worn
    f. Light is in place and waste receptacles (puncture-proof containers) available for needles and other sharps; hazardous materials bags available for contaminated disposables
    g. Receptacle used for soaking contaminated instruments so that blood will not dry
    h. Sterile transfer forceps used if it is necessary to move sterile items
        • Sides of container not covered with disinfecting solution must not be touched when removing forceps
        • Sterile gauze is used to wipe instrument dry after rinsing with sterile water

B. *Surgical instruments:* must be sterile if used invasively in the body

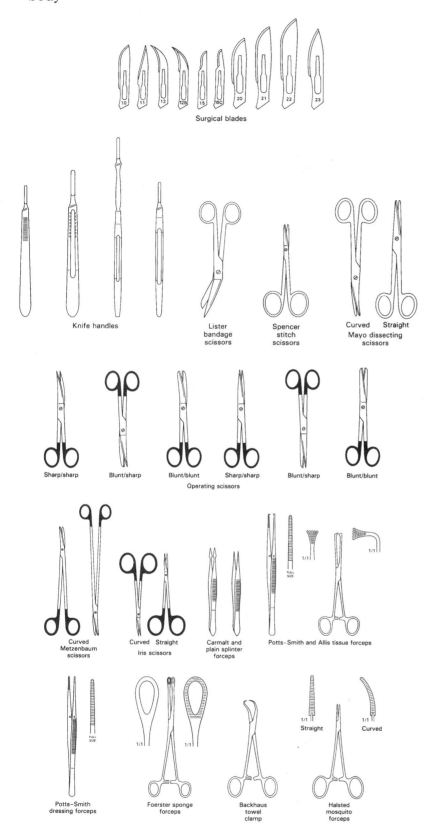

Surgical blades

Knife handles

Lister bandage scissors

Spencer stitch scissors

Curved   Straight
Mayo dissecting scissors

Sharp/sharp   Blunt/sharp   Blunt/blunt   Sharp/sharp   Blunt/sharp   Blunt/blunt
Operating scissors

Curved Metzenbaum scissors

Curved   Straight
Iris scissors

Carmalt and plain splinter forceps

Potts–Smith and Allis tissue forceps

Straight   Curved

Potts–Smith dressing forceps

Foerster sponge forceps

Backhaus towel clamp

Halsted mosquito forceps

Figure 14-2   Minor surgical instruments (Courtesy of the Miltex Instruments Co., Lake Success, NY).

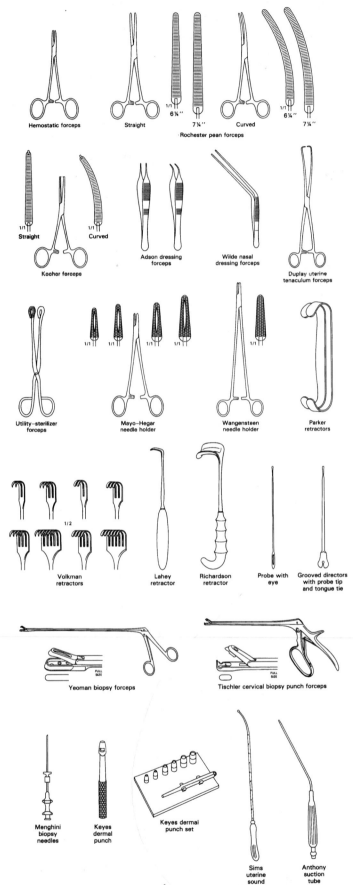

Figure 14-2 continued.

1. _Scissors:_ for cutting (may be sharp/sharp, sharp/blunt, blunt/blunt)
   a. _Iris scissors:_ small and sharp for precise cutting
   b. Straight or curved
   c. _Operative scissors:_ to cut tissue during surgery
   d. _Suture scissors:_ curved end helps get under sutures to cut them
2. _Forceps_
   a. _Splinter forceps:_ to remove splinters
   b. _Allis tissue forceps:_ grasping of delicate tissue
   c. _Sponge forceps:_ tips wrapped in gauze for blotting and sponging
   d. _Mosquito forceps:_ for clamping of very small vessels, and the like
   e. _Sterile transfer forceps:_ for moving sterile items
   f. _Hemostatic forceps:_ for clamping vessels
3. _Needle holders:_ clamp needle in place for suturing
   a. Sutures
      * _Absorbable:_ catgut
      * _Nonabsorbable:_ silk, cotton, polyester, nylon, and stainless steel
      * Size 11-0 (thin) to 7 (thick)
4. _Biopsy punch:_ punches out tissue for inspection under a microscope to see if it is normal
5. _Retractors:_ pull back muscles or wound edges
6. _Scalpel:_ sharp instrument for making incisions
7. _Cautery:_ seals off bleeders and helps coagulate blood

QUESTIONS

Match the definitions and the terms.

- a. Staphylococci
- b. Streptococci
- c. Diplococci
- d. Spirilla
- e. Bacilli
- f. Chlamydia
- g. Fungi
- h. Rickettsiae
- i. Protozoa
- j. Helminths
- k. Virus

_k_ 1. Smallest of all pathogenic microorganisms

_i_ 2. Single-celled animals, usually nonparasitic

_a_ 3. Round clusters of bacteria

_d_ 4. Spiral-shaped bacteria

_j_ 5. Parasitic worms

_b_ 6. Round bacteria in chains

_f_ 7. Small bacteria that cannot live without a host

_c_ 8. Round bacteria found in pairs

_h_ 9. Parasite causing spotted fever and typhus

_e_ 10. Rod-shaped bacteria

_g_ 11. Vegetative organisms, yeasts, and molds

Match the definitions and the terms.

- a. Sanitization
- b. Surgical asepsis
- c. Disinfection
- d. Medical asepsis

_d_ 12. Wash hands thoroughly; may leave on gold band ring

_b_ 13. Sterilization by autoclave

_a_ 14. Cleansing instruments with detergent

_d_ 15. Clean technique used during noninvasive procedures

_b_ 16. Sterile technique used during invasive procedures

_c_ 17. Rendering items as germ-free as possible by soaking in certain chemicals

_b_ 18. Scrub hands and forearms, and cleanse under fingernails for a prescribed amount of time

_b_ 19. No jewelry worn with this category of handwashing

Answers

1. **k** A virus is the smallest known pathogenic microorganism and can only be seen by using an electron microscope.

2. **i** Protozoa are single-celled animals that are usually nonparasitic.

3. **a** The morphology (size and shape) of staphylococci is round, and they are found in clusters.

4. **d** The bacteria spirilla are spiral-shaped.

5. **j** Helminths are microorganisms that are parasitic worms.

6. **b** Streptococci are round and found in chains.

7. **f** Chlamydia are small bacteria that cannot live without a host.

8. **c** Diplococci are round bacteria found in pairs.

9. **h** Rickettsiae are parasites known to cause spotted fever and typhus.

10. **e** Bacilli are rod-shaped bacteria.

11. **g** Fungi are vegetative organisms: for example, yeasts and molds.

12. **d** Medical asepsis is used when washing hands thoroughly before noninvasive procedures. A plain gold band ring can be worn during these types of procedures. Fingertips should be held downward.

13. **b** Surgical asepsis is used when autoclaving instruments. Autoclaving uses pressurized steam at, for example, 15 pounds of pressure at 250° F for 20 minutes (time, temperature, and pressure may vary). This renders instruments free of all pathogenic microorganisms, particularly spore-forming organisms.

14. **a** To sanitize instruments is to cleanse them with a detergent, just as one would wash dishes at home.

15. **d** Medical asepsis involves using clean technique during noninvasive procedures. Washing hands between patients is practicing medical asepsis.

16. **b** Surgical asepsis is used during invasive procedures. If the skin is broken or is going to be surgically incised, or if an instrument is going to be used past the normal body orifice, sterile instruments must be used and sterile technique must be practiced. This is called surgical asepsis.

17. **c** Soaking instruments or other items (such as rubber tubing) in a specified chemical can rid that item of most pathogenic organisms. This is called disinfection.

18. **b** Handwashing or scrubbing the hands and arms up to the elbows (while keeping fingertips pointed upward) for a certain amount of time according to strict protocol is using surgical asepsis. When scrubbing in this manner, one must remove all jewelry and clean under the fingernails as well.

19. **b** No jewelry is worn during surgical asepsis.

15

Clinical
Equipment

CHAPTER OUTLINE

Types of Equipment and Functions

I. TYPES OF EQUIPMENT AND FUNCTIONS

   A. *Thermometer:* for reading body temperature

      1. *Oral:* usually blue-tipped; has gradations of 0.2° F and ranges from approximately 94 to 106° F

         a. May be used under tongue or arm (reading will be 1° F lower than oral)

      2. *Rectal:* usually red-tipped with rounded bulb and same gradations as oral

         a. Inserted into rectal area (must be lubricated first) 1-½ inches for an adult, 1 inch for an infant (rectal temperature will be 1° F higher than oral)

      3. *Aural:* tympanic/ear thermometer resembles an otoscope; has disposable tips and is inserted into the ear for a few seconds until reading appears digitally (readings will be equivalent to oral)

      4. *Electronic thermometer:* usually has a disposable tip and can be used for oral, axillary, or rectal readings which will be displayed digitally

   B. *Sphygmomanometer (blood pressure cuff):* for obtaining blood pressure

      1. *Mercury:* has a vertical column of mercury for obtaining readings; gradations by 2 mmHg

      2. *Aneroid:* has a dial with a needle that points to numbers for readings; gradations by 2 mmHg

   C. *Stethoscope:* for auscultation (listening) to heart, lungs, bowel sounds, and arteries during blood pressure checks

   D. *Physician's scales:* for weighing patients

   E. *Microscope:* for identifying pathogenic microorganisms, counting blood cells and platelets, and urinary casts and crystals

   F. *Autoclave:* for sterilizing instruments by pressurized steam or gas

   G. *Ultrasonic cleaners:* to clean and disinfect instruments using chemicals and sound waves

   H. *Tape measure:* to measure head circumference of babies, pelvises of pregnant women, and so on

   I. *Glucometer:* to measure a patient's blood glucose

   J. *Autolet:* a device used to prick fingers quickly and almost painlessly for capillary blood samples

   K. *Defibrillator:* gives electrical shocks to the heart to set it back in rhythm and stop fibrillation

   L. *Audiometer:* machine for checking hearing; emits sounds of different levels for patient to identify

   M. *Otoscope:* device for looking into the ear

   N. *Snellen charts:* for checking distance visual acuity; Jaeger system for checking near visual acuity

   O. *Ophthalmoscope:* instrument for looking into a dilated eye to see the retina

P. *Tonometer:* measures pressure in the eye to check for glaucoma (always use ophthalmic anesthetic drops prior to using a tonometer)

Q. *Ishahara vision book:* has numbers made of dots of one color against dots of another color background for patient to identify to check color vision

R. *Electrocardiography (EKG) machine:* checks heart for arrythmias or irregularities

S. *Treadmill:* for stress testing a patient to see how much physical activity is appropriate and the heart's reaction to the stress

T. *Doppler:* instrument to magnify pulses and fetal heart sounds

U. *Spirometer:* measures lung capacity

V. *Sigmoidoscope:* scope that passes through the rectal area to the sigmoid colon to view the area for problems

W. *Wood's light:* purple fluorescent light used in dermatology to detect skin abnormalities

X. *Cast cutter:* cuts a cast to remove it from the patient's extremity; *cast spreader:* spreads the cast open after cutting it for removal

Y. *Cautery:* used to coagulate blood and to decrease capillary bleeding

Z. *Diathermy:* a form of heat to promote healing or reduce soreness of muscles

AA. *Centrifuge:* used to spin blood for hematocrits or urine for identification of casts and crystals; the formed elements will spin to the bottom and separate from the liquid portion

BB. *Hemoglobinometer:* determines the amount of hemoglobin in the blood

CC. *Hemacytometer:* used in counting blood cells

DD. *Ear irrigation syringe/equipment:* used to irrigate cerumen (wax) or foreign bodies from the ear

Match the definitions and the terms.

a. Defibrillator
b. Autolet
c. Glucometer
d. Doppler
e. Treadmill
f. Electrocardiography machine
g. Tonometer
h. Ishahara vision book
i. Snellen eye chart
j. Ophthalmoscope
k. Otoscope
l. Stethoscope

__f__ 1. Records electrical impulses from the heart

__e__ 2. Patient walks on this during stress testing

__a__ 3. Used to relay electrical impulses to the heart to regulate rhythm

__c__ 4. Tests blood sugar

__b__ 5. Assists in finger pricks for blood tests

__d__ 6. Magnifies the fetal heartbeat or other pulses throughout the body

__l__ 7. Used to listen to body sounds

__g__ 8. Measures eye pressure

__h__ 9. Checks color vision

__k__ 10. Enables the doctor to look inside the ear

__j__ 11. Enables the doctor to look inside the eye

__i__ 12. Helps measure distance visual acuity

Answers

1. **f** An EKG machine is attached to the patient by electrodes and leads. A lead is connected to electrodes on the fleshy part of each arm and the fleshy part of each leg. Precordial leads are also attached to electrodes placed around the left breast. These leads and electrodes register electrical impulses of the patient's heart and a recording is made.

2. **e** A treadmill is a rolling wide belt that patients walk while they are connected to an EKG machine. As the patient increases the speed of walking on this treadmill, the heart's activity is recorded.

3. **a** A defibrillator is a machine that delivers electrical impulses to the heart to stimulate a regular rhythm.

4. **c** After putting a drop of blood on a special strip, it will be inserted into a glucometer for a blood glucose reading.

5. **b** An autolet is a device used to prick fingers for blood tests such as the hematocrit and blood glucose.

6. **d** A Doppler is used for hearing fetal heart sounds at an early stage or for magnifying pulses to evaluate circulation.

7. **l** A stethoscope is used for auscultation or listening to body sounds from the heart, lungs, or bowels.

8. **g** A tonometer is used to measure eye pressure.

9. **h** The Ishahara method of screening for color blindness shows numbers made of colored dots against a background of dots of another color to check whether the patient can distinguish between the colors.

10. **k** An otoscope is used to look into the ear.

11. **j** An ophthalmoscope is used to look into the eye.

12. **i** The Snellen eye chart is used to check patients' distance vision.

16

Physician
Assisting

CHAPTER OUTLINE

Patient Preparation
Examination Techniques
Clinical Procedures

I. PATIENT PREPARATION

A. *Vital signs:* take and record all vital signs of each patient as a general rule

  1. *Temperature:* may be done electronically by ear, mouth, rectum, or axilla or manually by mouth, rectum, or axilla.

    a. Digital readings or 0.2° F increments on nonelectronic thermometers

      • Average range is 97 to 99° F (36.1 to 37.2° C)

    b. *Normal reading:* 98.6° F (add 1° F under the arm, subtract 1° F in the rectal area)

    c. *Afebrile:* no fever

  2. *Pulse:* usually taken at the radial artery (thumb side of the wrist area)

    a. Two to three fingers (but not the thumb) placed on the thumb side of the wrist

    b. Number of pulsations per minute counted (rate)

    c. Notation made as to whether or not rhythm is regular; notation is made as to volume type (weak, strong, bounding, thready)

    d. *Average range:* 60 to 100 beats/minute (varying with activity and body's physical condition)

    e. Types of arrythmias of the heart (thus, an abnormal pulse)

      • *Bradycardia:* slow heartbeat (less than 60 beats/minute)

      • *Tachycardia:* fast heartbeat (more than 100 beats/minute)

      • *Fibrillation:* quivering of the heart's muscle resulting in inadequate pumping of the heart's blood

  3. *Respirations:* after taking the pulse, one usually continues to hold the same position as for taking the pulse but looks at the patient's chest and counts breaths per minute

    a. One respiration equals one inhalation and one exhalation

    b. Shirt, back, or chest watched to notice breathing movements

    c. *Average range:* 12 to 25 breaths/minute

    d. Types of respirations

      • *Dyspnea:* difficulty in breathing

      • *Bradypnea:* abnormally slow breathing

      • *Tachypnea:* abnormally fast breathing

      • *Kussmaul's:* showing air hunger when breathing

      • *Cheyne-Stokes:* no breathing (apnea) followed by gradually increasing breaths

      • *Hyperpnea:* increased rate and depth in breathing

      • *Hypopnea:* decreased rate and depth in breathing

  4. *Blood pressure (BP):* sphygmomanometer and stethoscope needed; cuff goes around upper arm 1-½ to 2 inches above the elbow bend with cuff centered over brachial artery; the

stethoscope diaphragm is placed on the area of the brachial artery (not under the cuff)

    a. Blood pressure is the amount of pressure on the vessel walls as the heart pumps blood

    b. *Hypertension:* blood pressure readings consistently over 140/90

    c. *Hypotension:* if the patient is healthy, low BP is harmless

- *Orthostatic hypotension:* drop in BP due to sudden change from sitting to standing or from standing still for long periods
- *Shock:* a series of symptoms in which blood flow is inadequate for normal function; BP may be abnormally low or unobtainable

    d. Normal readings are below 140/90 with pulse pressure (difference between systolic, or top, reading, and diastolic, or bottom, reading) between 30 and 60

- Average pulse pressure = 40
- Abnormal pulse pressure = less than 30, more than 60

B. *Measurements* (also called mensurations)

    1. *Height:* can be checked by measuring rod attached to scales when patient stands on scales

    2. *Weight:* place a paper towel on scales; assist patient to scales and move weights until scale is balanced

    3. *Head circumference:* use tape measure to measure a baby's head

    4. *Visual acuity:* may use Snellen chart to check patient's distance vision

    5. *Spirometry:* used to check lung capacity

    6. *Urinalysis:* measure urine for color and other components

C. *Chief complaint:* patient's reason for an office visit

    1. Chief complaint must be known to prepare patient (e.g., if complaint is a sore throat, a strep test may be done and the patient asked to remove only clothing above the waist)

    2. Duration of complaint (how long has it been going on?)

    3. Medicines taken and whether they have helped

    4. What makes it better or worse?

    5. Other symptoms, together with chief complaint

    6. Other pertinent data, such as past history, surgical history, family history, and social history

II. EXAMINATION TECHNIQUES

A. Draping and positioning
1. _Supine:_ flat on the back with the legs straight

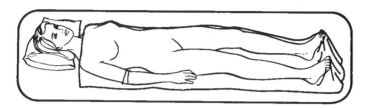

Figure 16-1A Horizontal recumbent position.

    a. _Drape:_ rectangular drape up to the chin
    b. Appropriate for examining any anterior area (on the front of the body)
2. _Dorsal recumbent:_ flat on the back with the knees bent

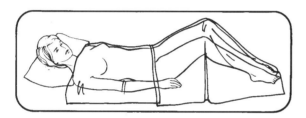

Figure 16-1B Dorsal recumbent position.

    a. _Drape:_ rectangular or diamond-shaped with lower point of the drape between the knees
    b. Abdominal muscles are relaxed; therefore, position is good for an abdominal examination
    c. Rectal or vaginal areas can be examined
3. _Lithotomy:_ flat on the back with the knees bent and in stirrups

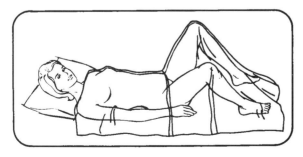

Figure 16-1C Lithotomy position.

a. *Drape:* rectangular or diamond-shaped
  - *Diamond-shaped:* pointed flap may be lifted for examination
  - *Rectangular:* lower portion of the sheet is between the lower legs; it may be pushed upward with both of the assistant's hands and wrapped around the legs but out of the way of the examination area
b. Appropriate for examination of female vaginal area, taking Pap smears, and so on
4. *Prone:* on the stomach with the head to the side

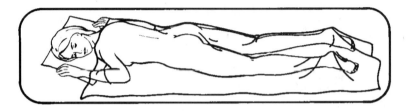

Figure 16-1D Prone position.

a. *Drape:* rectangular
b. Appropriate for examination of the dorsal side of the body (backside)
5. *Right or left Sims:* on the right or left side with the lower leg slightly bent and the top leg sharply flexed

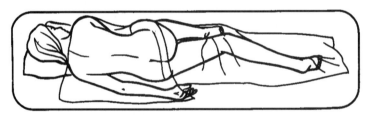

Figure 16-1E Left Sims position.

a. *Drape:* diamond-shaped drape with pointed end or flap over area to be examined, usually the rectal area
b. *Left Sims:* position for taking rectal temperatures or giving enemas

6. _Trendelenburg:_ on the back with the head lower than the feet

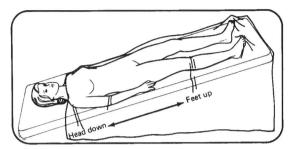

Figure 16-1F Trendelenburg position.

    a. Rectangular drape
    b. Position for fainting (syncope) or shock recovery (unless head or chest injury)

7. _Fowlers:_ sitting position

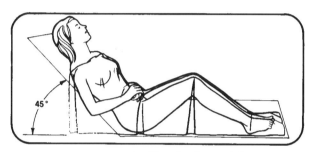

Figure 16-1G Fowler's position.

    a. Patient is gowned, then a drape placed across the lap
    b. Appropriate for examining the throat, lungs, or any area above the waist; possibly the legs and reflexes

8. _Knee—chest:_ on knees and chest with buttocks in the air

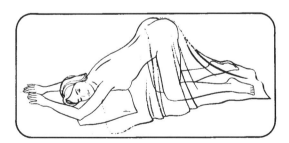

Figure 16-1H Knee—chest position.

    a. _Drape:_ diamond-shaped drape so that pointed end is at the feet and can be lifted for examination
    b. Appropriate for rectal examination, rigid sigmoidoscopy, and prolapsed uterus

B. Methods of examination
1. *Inspection:* generally looking the patient over
    a. Notations made of any deformities, unusual mannerisms, general health of the body, posture, and use of the extremities (arms and legs)
2. *Palpation:* examining by feeling specific areas of the body
    a. For example, breast examinations would be done by palpation
    b. *Bimanual:* using both hands, as in feeling the ovaries
    c. *Digital:* using one finger, as in rectal examinations
3. *Percussion:* tapping directly on an area or putting the fingers on an area and tapping the fingers
    a. *Use:* to discern outlines of organs to check for enlargement
    b. Appropriate for checking fluid-filled areas
    c. *Reflexes:* checked by percussion hammer or reflex hammer
4. *Auscultation:* listening to body sounds
    a. Lungs listened to symmetrically to compare one side to the other
    b. Auscultation of bowels may reveal a blockage or impaction
    c. Heart and pulse sounds may detect abnormalities in rhythm, for example
5. Mensuration (measuring)
    a. Height and weight
    b. Head circumference of babies
    c. Chest circumference
    d. Pelvic measurements
    e. Length of extremities, angles of joints
    f. Fat measurements
6. *Manipulation:* movement of an area, especially the joints
    a. Detection of the amount of movement in a joint or its range of motion

III. CLINICAL PROCEDURES

All procedures should be explained to the patient prior to performing them to alleviate the patient's anxiety. Hands should always be washed before and after each procedure. Universal precautions should always be followed using barriers (gloves, masks, etc.) appropriate to the procedure. Record all procedures in the patient's chart.

A. *Tine test:* screening test for tuberculosis
1. Inside of forearm is cleansed with antiseptic from inside out
2. Cap of tine test is removed and tines are pressed firmly while pulling the skin taut
3. Site of the test is recorded
4. Area observed after 48 to 72 hours and results recorded

B. _Scratch test_: allergy determination (tests may be invalid if the patient is taking antihistamine)
   1. Site is cleansed (usually on the inside of the forearm or on the patient's back)
   2. Identification of each area, leaving approximately 2 inches between sites
   3. Each site is scratched with a separate sterile sharp instrument and a drop of allergen is added to the site
   4. Observation of reaction (within 30 minutes) and results recorded
   5. Site is cleansed
C. Patch test
   1. Site is cleansed (usually on the inside forearm or on the patient's back)
   2. Identification of each area, leaving approximately 2 inches between sites
   3. Drop of allergen to each area with a cellophane adhesive patch covering or application of a gauze square impregnated with suspected allergen
   4. Site is checked in 48 hours and results recorded
D. Pelvic exam
   1. Patient in lithotomy position (in stirrups)
   2. Vaginal speculum warmed with warm water or light warming tray unless sterility is needed
   3. Doctor is given needed instruments (cytology brush, cervical spatula)
   4. Microscopic slides for Pap test are smeared in correct area (V = vaginal, C = cervical, E = endocervical)
   5. Fixative is sprayed on slides
   6. Lubricant is transferred to the doctor's glove for a bimanual and rectal exam
   7. Test for occult blood is prepared
   8. Slides and the occult blood test are labeled
E. Visual acuity for distance
   1. Vision of right eye tested first; therefore, the patient will put cover in front of the left eye so that the eye underneath the cover is open but not mashed
   2. Indicate line on Snellen chart the patient is to read
   3. Patient will stand back 20 feet and continue reading smaller lines until letters are missed
   4. Record the smallest line read, indicating how many letters were missed (if the 20/30 line was read but the patient missed two, write 20/30 -2)
   5. Left eye: same procedure

F. Irrigating eyes and ears
   1. Outside area is washed (auricle/pinna for the ear, eyelids for the eye)
   2. Patient holds the drainage basin and towel under the ear while flow is directed toward the upper ear canal or beside the eye so that the flow will be from the inner to outer canthus of the eye
   3. Observe the area to be irrigated to identify material to be irrigated
   4. Irrigate with a steady stream of liquid until all material is washed out
   5. Ear/eye is wiped dry and procedure is recorded
      a. Ear of an adult is pulled upward and back
      b. Ear of a child is pulled down and back
      c. Eye is held open gently or upper and lower lids are rolled back with cotton-tipped applicators
G. Infant head circumference
   1. Tape is placed around the head at an area right above ears and at eyebrows
   2. Tape is pulled snug and measurement is recorded to nearest 0.01 cm
H. Bandaging and applying dressings
   1. Protocol or orders are followed as to antiseptic application
   2. Sterile dressing is applied to cover the wound adequately
   3. Area is bandaged securely extending 1 to 2 inches above and below the dressing and taped as needed (may use tubular bandage for fingers, etc.)
   4. Record is made of how the area looked, exact steps followed, and supplies used
   5. Removal of old dressings and bandages: always cut through the bandage on the area opposite the wound site and record the amount and appearance of drainage
   6. Tape is always pulled toward the wound
I. Removing staples and sutures
   1. Area is cleansed
   2. Staple remover is inserted under each staple and pressed together
   3. Sutures: grasp each knot with forceps and cut the suture as close to the skin as possible to prevent drawing contaminated suture through the skin; suture should slip out easily
   4. Staples or sutures should be counted to be sure all have been removed
   5. Dress the area if necessary and record the procedure
J. Application of a hot or cold compress
   1. Compress is never applied directly to the skin; there should be toweling between the compress and skin, or if the wound is open, use sterile compresses or towels
   2. Temperature of the compress is checked before applying so as not to burn the patient

3. Compress is left for the prescribed amount of time, but the patient is consulted as to comfort

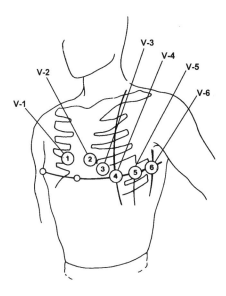

Figure 16-2 Precordial chest lead placement.

K. Performing an EKG
   1. Preparation of the skin by rubbing the area briskly, applying gel, if needed, for better conduction, and attaching the electrodes to the following areas:
      a. Inside area of the right upper arm
      b. Inside area of the left upper arm
      c. Inside area of the right lower leg
      d. Inside area of the left lower leg
      e. Areas for chest or precordial leads
         • *V-1*: right of sternum at the fourth intercostal space
         • *V-2*: left of sternum at the fourth intercostal space
         • *V-3*: halfway between leads V2 and V4
         • *V-4*: midclavicular line at the fifth intercostal space
         • *V-5*: fifth intercostal space halfway between leads V4 and V6
         • *V-6*: horizontal to lead V5, but midaxillary under the left arm
   2. Appropriate leads are attached to the electrodes
      a. Standard or bipolar leads
         • *Lead I*: electrical activity between the right arm and left arm
         • *Lead II*: electrical activity between the right arm and left leg
         • *Lead III*: electrical activity between the left arm and left leg

   b. Augmented or unipolar leads
- *Lead AVR (augmented voltage, right arm):* electrical activity from the midpoint between the left arm and left leg, to the right arm
- *Lead AVL (augmented voltage, left arm):* electrical activity from the midpoint between the right arm and left leg, to the left arm
- *Lead AVF (augmented voltage, foot):* electrical activity from the midpoint between the right arm and left arm, to the left leg

   c. Chest or precordial leads (see leads V1-V6)
3. Standardization of the machine
4. Automatic mode for EKG is used or dials are set to each lead setting and each is run separately
5. Artifacts (interferences with recording of EKG) are corrected
6. Markings are made in areas of any unusual occurrences that change recording, such as the patient moving or coughing; re-record when the patient is settled
7. *Paper:* heat sensitive

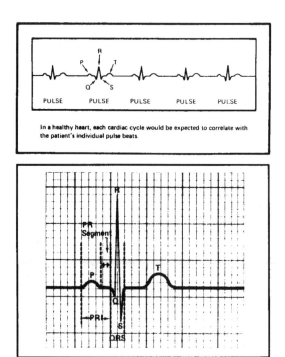

Figure 16-3 EKG recordings.

   a. Smallest block: 1 mm x 1mm; representing 0.02 second
   b. 300 blocks = 6-second strip
8. *Tracings:* P, QRS, T waves
   a. P wave: atrial contraction; indication that the SA node is working
   b. QRS: ventricular contraction

L. Body mechanics
   1. Push, don't pull
   2. Work area should be at or a little above waist level
   3. Items should be carried as close to the body as possible
   4. Stoop rather than bend
   5. Stepping stool should be used rather than reaching
   6. Correct patient transfer methods should be used
M. Catheterization
   1. Urinary drainage of bladder
   2. Method for obtaining sterile specimens
   3. Irrigation or instillation of medicines into bladder
   4. Procedure should be sterile
      a. Wipe each side of the labia with indicated antiseptic, then wipe the middle
      b. Insert catheter until fluid drainage is observed
      c. Obtain specimen, or attach tubing to bag if indwelling

QUESTIONS

Explain what is wrong in each of the following examples

1. A patient's vital signs are recorded as T 98.6, P 14, R 70, BP 120/90.
2. A patient's vital signs are T 98.6, P 75, R 12, BP 150/100.
3. A patient's vital signs are T 104, P 80, R 12, BP 100/60.
4. A medical assistant is checking a patient's pulse by placing the thumb over the radial artery on the left wrist.
5. A patient's heart rate is 50. _Brady_
6. A patient's heart rate is 110. _↑ tachy_
7. A medical assistant recorded a patient's respirations as 28. The patient is, however, breathing normally at 14 breaths/minute.
8. A patient has a period of no breathing, then gradually begins to breathe faster with each breath. _ch/st_
9. A patient is asked to remove all of his clothes. His chief complaint is sore throat. _↑OP_
10. A patient in shock is placed in the Fowler's position.
11. A vomiting patient is placed in the supine position.

Match the word and the definition.
a. Prone
b. Supine
c. Left Sims
d. Knee-chest
e. Lithotomy
f. Trendelenburg
g. Fowler's
h. Dorsal recumbent

_b_ 12. Flat on the back, the legs straight
_h g_ 13. Flat on the back, the knees bent
_e_ 14. Feet in stirrups, flat on the back, female pelvic examination position
_a_ 15. On the stomach, the head to side
_c_ 16. On the left side, the left leg slightly bent, the right leg sharply bent
_f_ 17. Head lower than the feet

_d_ 18. On knees and chest, with the buttocks in the air
_g_ 19. Sitting

a. Inspection
b. Palpation
c. Percussion
d. Auscultation
e. Mensuration
f. Manipulation

_e_ 20. The act of measuring
_b_ 21. Examining by touch
_f_ 22. Movement of the joints
_a_ 23. Looking the patient over
_c_ 24. Tapping
_d_ 25. Listening
_e_ 26. Head circumference
_a_ 27. Looking at the patient's gait (method of walking)
_b_ 28. Breast examination
_d_ 29. Checking for bowel sounds
_f_ 30. Flexing the arm at the elbow
_c_ 31. Tapping around the area of the liver to detect its outline

True—False

_F_ 32. A tine test determines a patient's allergies.
_F_ 33. When determining allergies by the scratch test method, the medical assistant should perform each allergen test as close to the previous one as possible.
_F_ 34. A fixative should never be sprayed on Pap smears.
_T_ 35. A patient missed one letter on the 20/20 line. This should be recorded as 20/20-1.
_F_ 36. Head circumference should be measured from the chin to the top of the head.
_F_ 37. A bandage should be removed by cutting across the wound above the dressing.

132   *Chapter 16*   **Physician Assisting**

_F_ 38. Hot compresses should be applied directly to the skin for maximal effect.

_F_ 39. The V-1 lead is placed at the fifth inter-costal space at the right of the ster-num.

_T_ 40. The V-2 lead is placed at the fourth intercostal space at the left of the sternum.

Answers

1. The pulse was recorded as 14 and respira-tions were recorded as 70. Normal pulse is between 60 and 80 beats per minute and normal respirations are between 12 and 16 per minute. In this case, pulse and respirations were probably interchanged.

2. Blood pressure over 140/90 on more than one occasion may be considered hypertension. Normal blood pressure is usually below 140/90.

3. Normal temperature is 98.6. In this case, a temperature of 104 is very high.

4. Pulse should be taken by placing two to three fingers (but not the thumb since the thumb has a pulse) on the radial artery on the wrist of either arm.

5. A patient's heart rate of 50 is considered too low unless the patient is very athletic. A rate of 50 is called bradycardia.

6. A heart rate of 110 is above normal. This rate is called tachycardia.

7. One respiration equals one inhalation and one exhalation. If a patient is breathing normally, but the chart reads R 28, the assistant must have counted each inhala-tion and each exhalation, thus doubling the respiration rate.

8. A period of no breathing, then increasing-ly faster breathing is called Cheyne—Stokes breathing. This is an abnormal breathing rate.

9. A patient should not have to remove all of his/her clothes to be checked for a sore throat. A medical assistant should be familiar with the doctor's methods of examination so as not to subject the patient to unnecessary removal of cloth-ing.

10. A patient in shock should be placed with the head lower than the feet. This is called the Trendelenburg position. If there is a head or chest injury, this posi-tion is contraindicated.

11. A vomiting patient should never be placed in the supine position. A vomiting patient should be placed on his/her side. The prone or the supine position could cause the patient to aspirate his/her own vomi-tus and thus choke or get aspiration pneumonia.

12. b Supine is flat on the back with the legs straight.

13. h Dorsal recumbent is flat on the back with the knees bent.

14. e The lithotomy position: the female patient's feet are placed in stirrups in readiness for the pelvic examination.

15. a Prone is on the stomach with the head to the side.

16. c Left Sims: the patient is on the left side with the left leg slightly bent and the right leg flexed sharply.

17. f Trendelenburg: the patient's head is lower than the feet.

18. d The knee—chest position: the patient is on the knees with the buttocks in the air.

19. g Fowler's position is a sitting position.

20. e Mensuration is the act of measuring.

21. b Examining by feeling is palpation.

22. f Manipulation is movement of the joints.

23. a Inspection is the act of looking the patient over.

24. c Percussion is the act of tapping.

25. d Auscultation is the act of listening.

26. e Head circumference is a measurement, thus mensuration.

27. a Looking at the patient's gait or the way she/he walks is called inspection.

28. b The doctor palpates or feels for lumps in the breast during a breast examination.

29. d When listening to the abdominal area for sounds, the doctor is auscultating for bowel sounds.

30. f Manipulation is being done when the doc-tor flexes the patient's arm at the elbow.

31. c Percussion is taking place when the doc-tor taps around the area of the liver to detect its outline.

32. False A tine test screens for tuberculosis.

33. False Each area for a scratch test should be approximately 2 inches apart for valid results.

34. **False** A fixative is always applied on Pap smears.
35. **True**
36. **False** Head circumference is measured around the infant's head at the eyebrows and just above the ears.
37. **False** Remove a bandage by cutting through the bandage on the side opposite the wound.
38. **False** Hot compresses should never be applied directly to the skin, due to possible burns.

There should be a towel or layers of toweling between the patient's skin and the compress.
39. **False** The V-1 lead should be placed at the right of the sternum at the fourth intercostal space.
40. **True**

17

Laboratory Procedures

CHAPTER OUTLINE

Laboratory Tests
Specimen Collection
Normal Laboratory Values
Laboratory Safety
Microscope Use

I. LABORATORY TESTS

   A. *Urinalysis:* collection and testing of urine
      1. Physical examination of urine
         a. *Odor*
            • *Foul odor:* infection
            • *Fruity odor:* diabetes
            • *Ammonia odor:* urine that has been at room temperature for a while or has a high concentration of bacteria
         b. *Color:* normal is pale to dark yellow
            • *Red:* hematuria (urine with blood); some foods or drugs may cause redness
            • *Brownish:* bilirubin, bile, or melanin in the urine
         c. *Transparency:* clear is normal
            • *Cloudy:* may have bacteria or excessive amounts of red blood cells, white blood cells, or other components; may become cloudy after standing at room temperature
         d. *Specific gravity:* ratio of the weight of a certain amount of urine as compared to the same amount of distilled water
      2. Chemical examination of urine
         a. *Reagent strips:* dipped into the urine specimen and read by color changes in specified amounts of time
            • *pH (acidity or alkalinity):* below 7 = acid; above 7 = alkaline; 5.5 to 8 = average
            • *Protein:* negative to trace = normal
            • *Glucose:* negative = normal
            • *Ketones:* negative = normal
            • *Bilirubin:* negative = normal
            • *Blood:* negative = normal
            • *Urobilinogen:* 0.1 to 1.0 Ehrlich unit/dl = normal
         b. Confirmatory tests
            • *Protein:* treat urine with an acid to cause protein to precipitate; indicates protein in urine
            • *Sugars:* Clinitest tablet is the most common; tablet is dropped in urine and reacts if positive (Caution: may have false-positive results)
            • *Glucose tolerance test:* confirmatory for glucose
            • *Ketones:* Acetest tablet dropped in urine changes color if positive
            • *Bilirubin:* Icotest; color changes when tablet dropped on a urine-soaked pad if positive
      3. *Urine sediment:* microscopic examination of urine (after centrifuging and pouring off the clear portion, called supernatant)
         a. *Red blood cells:* indicate trauma or disease (possibly contamination if patient is a female having menses); normal is 1 to 2 (use the high-power lens on the microscope)

b. *White blood cells:* indicate infection; normal is less than 5 (use the high-power lens on the microscope)

c. *Epithelial cells:* probably normal unless high number present from the kidneys; normal is 1 to 2 (use the low-power lens on the microscope)

d. *Bacteria:* indicate infection and are abnormal (high power)

e. *Yeasts or protozoa:* indicate disease and are abnormal (high power)

f. *Hyaline casts:* usually normal (low power)

g. Granular or cellular casts may indicate disease (low power)

h. Amorphous urate, uric acid, and calcium oxalate crystals are normal in acid urine (high power)

i. Amorphous phosphate, triple phosphate, and calcium carbonate crystals are normal in alkaline urine (high power)

j. Cystine, tyrosine, leucine, cholesterol, and sulfonamide crystals are abnormal (high power)

B. Hematology

1. *Hematocrit:* volume of red blood cells in a specific volume of blood

    a. *Low:* anemia or abnormal bleeding

    b. *High:* dehydration or polycythemia vera

    c. Performance of a microhematocrit test

    • Two heparinized capillary tubes of blood are collected

    • Tubes are placed in a centrifuge directly across from each other and with the sealed end against the gasket toward the outside edge of the centrifuge

    • Centrifuge is run with locked lid

    • Tubes are placed on a microhematocrit reader and averaged

    • Results are recorded

2. *Hemoglobin:* oxygen-carrying component of red blood cells

    a. Hemoglobin is one-third of hematocrit

    b. *Hemoglobinometer:* use with capillary puncture to determine the amount of hemoglobin in blood

3. *Erythrocyte sedimentation rate:* speed at which red blood cells settle

    a. Normal rate is slow: 1 mm every 5 minutes

    b. Abnormal rate is indicative of inflammation

    c. Performance of a sedimentation rate test

    • Venous blood is collected into a tube with an anticoagulant (a lavendar-colored stopper is used)

    • Tube is placed into a rack for 1 hour

    • Distance the erythrocytes have fallen is measured and recorded

    • Amount of blood and tube size varies with method of testing

4. _Red cell count:_ estimate of the number of circulating red blood cells
   a. Increase indicates erythrocytosis
      • Polycythemia vera is an example
      • People living at high altitudes may have increased cell counts
   b. Decrease indicates erythrocytopenia
      • Usually, anemias are an example
   c. Manual red blood cell counting
      • Red cells are mixed with a diluting fluid
      • Hemacytometer (a glass slide made specifically with grids for counting blood cells) is filled
      • Cells are counted; first row, left to right, second row, right to left, and so on, on side 1 of the hemacytometer
      • Cells are counted only in four corner squares and center square of the large middle square of the hemacytometer
      • Cells touching the lower or right edge of each square are not counted
      • Findings are recorded; then side 2 of the hemacytometer is counted and recorded, the two sides averaged, and four zeros are added to the average
5. _White cell counting:_ estimate of the number of circulating white blood cells
   a. Increase indicates leukocytosis
      • Infections cause an increase
      • Increase expected with leukemia
   b. Decrease indicates leukopenia
      • Chemotherapy may cause a decrease
      • Decrease expected with radiation
   c. Types of white blood cells
      • _Neutrophils:_ ingest bacteria
      • _Eosinophils:_ aid during allergic reactions
      • _Basophils:_ may absorb blood clots
      • _Monocytes:_ aid in immunity and during infection
      • _Lymphocytes:_ B cells produce antibodies; T cells help immunity
   d. Manual white cell counting

neu

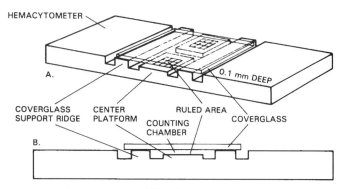

Figure 17-1 The hemacytometer.

- Blood is mixed with white cell diluting fluid
- Hemacytometer is filled
- Cells within the four large corner squares are counted in the same manner and using the same boundary method as that used for RBCs

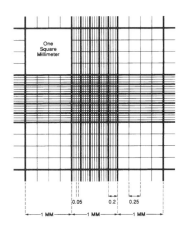

Figure 17-2 The hemacytometer has ruled areas for cell counting.

- Cells from sides 1 and 2 are counted and averaged, and multiplied by 50

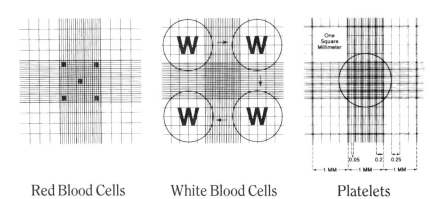

Red Blood Cells   White Blood Cells   Platelets

Figure 17-3 Areas for counting each type of blood cell.

6. _Platelet counting:_ estimate of circulating platelets
   a. Increase indicates thrombocytosis
      • Increase appears after a splenectomy
      • Increase expected with polycythemia vera
   b. Decrease indicates thrombocytopenia
      • Chemotherapy may cause a decrease
      • Radiation may cause a decrease
   c. Manual platelet count
      • Blood and diluting fluid for platelets are mixed
      • Hemacytometer is filled
      • Platelets in the entire center are counted, using the same counting method and same boundary method as that used for RBC and WBC counting
      • Two sides are counted and averaged, then multiplied by 1000
7. _Blood smears:_ for viewing blood components under microscope
   a. Small drop of blood is added to a clean slide near the end
   b. Another slide is used to pull back into the drop of blood until it spreads along the edges of the slide
   c. Second slide (that is in the drop of blood) is pushed forward to smear blood
   d. First slide is then dried, fixed, and stained
8. _Staining blood smears:_ components of the blood may be seen better
   a. Slide is placed on staining rack with drainage system underneath
   b. Blood smear is flooded with Wright's stain and left standing
   c. Buffer is added and left standing
   d. Slide is rinsed gently and placed on end to dry
   e. Instructions are always followed for times (some quick stains can be dipped and rinsed in a very short time)
9. _Differential white blood cell (leukocyte) count:_ finding percentages of each of the five types of white blood cells
   a. One drop of immersion oil is used; view under microscope the area of the stained blood smear where red cells barely touch
   b. Count 100 total cells using a pattern of moving down, then to the right, moving up, then to the right, then down again, and so on
   c. Record each type of leukocyte (white cell)
   d. Observe morphology (size and shape) and number of red cells and record observations
   e. Observe morphology and number of platelets and record
10. _Bleeding time:_ evaluates blood's ability to clot
   a. Standard-sized incision is made
   b. Amount of time it takes to stop bleeding is timed and recorded

11. _ABO slide typing:_ determination of blood types
    a. Microscopic slide is marked as side A and side B
    b. Anti-A serum is dropped on the A side and anti-B serum on the B side
    c. Blood is dropped on each side and stirred with separate stirrers
    d. If agglutination (clumping) occurs on side labeled A, then blood type is A
    e. Agglutination on B side = blood type B
    f. Agglutination on both sides = blood type AB
    g. No agglutination on either side = blood type O
C. Bacteriology
    1. Preparing a bacteriological smear
        a. Swab method
            • Swab of bacterial specimen is rolled onto a microscopic slide
            • Slide is air dried
            • Slide is passed through the flame of a bunsen burner
            • Slide is stained
        b. Culture tube or petri dish method
            • Inoculating loop is passed through the flame and a drop or two of water is added to the slide
            • Loop is reflamed
            • Loop is touched to bacteria, being careful not to touch the edges of the tube or petri dish, and bacteria is spread around in water on the slide
            • Slide is allowed to air dry, then is passed through the flame to heat fix
    2. _Gram staining:_ applying dye to bacteria for easier identification
        a. Slide is placed on staining rack with drainage system underneath
        b. Slide is flooded with crystal violet dye
        c. Slide is rinsed gently with water
        d. Slide is flooded with mordant (Gram's iodine), which causes the dye to adhere
        e. Slide is rinsed gently with water
        f. Decolorizer is added until clear (usually happens quickly)
        g. Slide is rinsed gently with water
        h. Slide is counterstained with safranin (red dye)
        i. Slide is rinsed gently with water
        j. Slide is blotted or air dried
        k. Oil immersion objective is used to view
        l. Purple = gram positive
        m. Pinkish red = gram negative

D. Occult blood
  1. Patient preparation and instructions for diet are necessary for accurate results and quality control
  2. Specimen is obtained and smeared on the testing area
  3. Reagent is added according to manufacturer's instructions
  4. Positive or negative result is read and recorded

II. SPECIMEN COLLECTION

For all blood and body fluid collections, UNIVERSAL PRECAUTIONS MUST BE USED; hands are always washed before and after each procedure, gloves and other appropriate barriers are used, all hazardous waste is disposed of in a BIOHAZARD (red-labeled bag) container, and all sharps are disposed of in a puncture-proof container! Refrain from direct patient contact if you have open or exudative lesions.

  A. *Urine:* first void in the morning is the most concentrated, and therefore is the best specimen for concentrated tests; refrigerate if not tested right away, or a fresh specimen may be obtained in office

     1. *Midstream:* patient lets first few seconds of urination pass into toilet, then begins to urinate in specimen container
     2. *Clean-catch:* used to determine if bacteria are present
        a. Area around the urethral opening is retracted
        b. Males wipe urethral opening three separate times using three separate towelettes
        c. Females wipe each side of urethral opening using separate towelettes, then front to back across urethral opening
        d. Urination begins, and midstream urine is collected

  B. *Capillary puncture* (finger, earlobe, or heel stick)

     1. Site is cleansed with alcohol and dried with sterile gauze
     2. Skin is held taut and lanced quickly
     3. First drop of blood is wiped away
     4. Capillary tube (heparinized) is filled two-thirds full, holding it horizontally
     5. Clean end of tube is placed in sealing clay
     6. Pressure is applied to the puncture site to stop bleeding

  C. *Venipuncture:* collection of blood from a vein (usually the median cephalic vein of the forearm)

     1. Site is cleansed with alcohol using circular, inside-out method
     2. Tourniquet is applied around mid-upper arm (not so tight that the pulse cannot be felt and for no more than 2 minutes)
     3. Skin is held taut; needle (20 to 22 gauge) is inserted bevel up into the vein
     4. Plunger is pulled back to aspirate blood or if using Vacutainer method, tube is pushed up into Vacutainer holder unit but not punctured far enough to release vacuum until appropriately positioned in vein
     5. Tourniquet is released before removing the needle
     6. Needle is removed and pressure is applied to the site

D. Collection tubes for blood
  1. _Red:_ no anticoagulant so serum will separate for testing purposes
  2. _Purple:_ EDTA (an anticoagulant) is used for hematology studies using unclotted blood (smears)
  3. _Green:_ for heparinized tests of unclotted blood other than smears
  4. _Blue:_ sodium citrate for coagulation tests
E. _Stool collection:_ check feces for parasites or occult blood
  1. Paper drape or cellophane wrap placed under toilet seat to catch stool or the doctor may digitally examine patient and use stool sample from gloved finger
  2. Wooden stick is used to obtain sample of stool to smear on testing area (if occult blood)
  3. Wooden stick or gloved hands may be used to obtain sample for collection tube for other testing, such as for parasites
F. Throat swabbing
  1. Patient is asked to open mouth and say "ah"
  2. Tongue depressor is used to keep tongue out of the way while rolling sterile swab on both sides of the throat
  3. Specimen is applied to culture medium or inserted into a culturette tube and labeled
G. Sputum collection
  1. Best specimen is the first morning collection
  2. Deep breath and productive cough are needed for deep lung secretions
  3. Collection container should be sterile

III. NORMAL LABORATORY VALUES
  A. Urine
    1. Volume = 750—2000 ml/24 hours
    2. Color = yellow
    3. Transparency = clear
    4. Specific gravity = 1.005—1.030 (stated as "ten o five to ten thirty)
    5. Protein, glucose, ketones, bilirubin, blood, urobilinogen, bacteria, red blood cells are all negative
    6. White blood cells = 0 to 4
    7. Occasional epithelial cells
    8. Occasional hyaline casts
    9. Only cystine, leucine, tyrosine, and cholesterol crystals are reportably significant
    10. pH = 4 to 8
  B. Hematology
    1. Red blood cells = 4,000,000 to 6,000,000 per mm^3
    2. White blood cells = 4,000 to 11,000 per mm^3

3. Platelets = 150,000 to 400,000 per mm^3
4. Neutrophils = 50—60%
5. Eosinophils = 1—3%
6. Basophils = 0—1%
7. Monocytes = 3—8%
8. Lymphocytes = 25—40%
9. Hematocrit = 40—50%, males; 35—45%, females
10. Hemoglobin = 13—17 g/dl, males; 12—15 g/dl, females
    (*Note:* Hemoglobin is always one-third of hematocrit)
11. Bleeding time = 1—8 minutes
12. Sedimentation rate = 0—20 mm/hour (depending on the method used)
13. Occult blood or parasites = none should be found
14. Cholesterol = <200 mg/dl (LDL=60—180 mg/dl, HDL = 30—80 mg/dl)
15. Triglycerides = 40—150 mg/dl
16. Glucose = 70—115 mg/dl (fasting, serum)
17. BUN (blood urea nitrogen) = 9—25 mg/ml

IV. LABORATORY SAFETY

A. No eating or drinking in the laboratory

B. Laboratory jacket and closed-toed shoes are always worn

C. Universal Precautions are always followed

D. Work area is cleaned before and after each procedure (10 percent household bleach such as Clorox solution often used because it kills the AIDS virus on contact)

E. Hands are washed before and after each laboratory procedure

F. Safety glasses are worn as needed

G. Needle sticks or other incidents are reported promptly

H. Laboratories are equipped with safety devices such as a fire blanket, eye-rinsing station, fire extinguishers, safety glasses, and a body-wash station

I. Biohazard containers are provided for hazardous wastes; puncture-proof containers for sharps

J. All OSHA (Occupational Safety and Health Act) and CLIA (Clinical Laboratory Improvement Amendments) rules are followed

K. All MSDS (Material Safety Data Sheets) are read and filed

V. MICROSCOPE USE

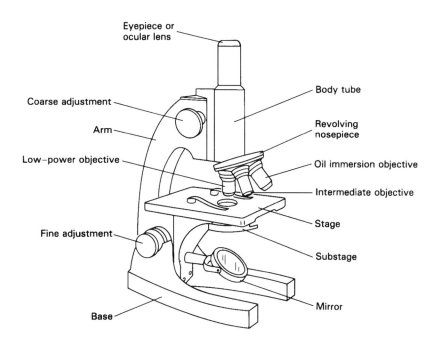

Figure 17-4 The microscope.

A. *Three objectives* (magnifying lenses)
   1. Low is magnified 10 times
   2. High is magnified 40, 43, or 45 times
   3. Oil immersion is magnified 95, 97, or 100 times
B. *Oculars:* 10x, 15x, and 20x
C. *Stage:* part on which slides are placed
D. *Condenser:* directs available light
E. *Diaphragm:* regulates amount of light
F. Adjustments for focus
   1. *Coarse:* for low power only (after focusing with low power, other powers can be rotated into place; then use only the fine adjustment or slides will be broken)
   2. *Fine:* used after object is initially found; clears image

True—False

_F_ 1. Physical examination of urine consists of looking at color only.

_T_ 2. Urine can be examined chemically by dipping reagent strips into the urine and noting color changes in specified amounts of time.

_F_ 3. Specific gravity is expressed as a ratio of an amount of urine to a specific amount of blood.

_F_ 4. Cholesterol crystals found in urine are normal.

_T_ 5. Increased white blood cells found in urine are usually indicative of infection.

_F_ 6. Hematocrit is found by taking one-third of hemoglobin.

_T_ 7. An abnormal sedimentation rate is usually indicative of inflammation.

_T_ 8. All blood cells may be decreased after chemotherapy or radiation treatments.

_T_ 9. Blood smears are stained so that components of blood can be seen better.

_T_ 10. If clumping or agglutination occurs on side A when testing for blood types, the blood type is A.

X _T_ 11. A mordant causes dye to demolish bacterial walls.

_F_ 12. Safranin dyes the cell walls purple.

_F_ 13. The last urine voided in the evening is the best specimen for urinalysis.

_F_ 14. Capillary puncture is done at the median cephalic vein.

_T_ 15. Always cleanse sites of puncture or injections in a circular motion from the inside out.

_T_ 16. EDTA and heparin are anticoagulants.

_F_ 17. Laboratory jacket and open-toed shoes must be worn in the laboratory at all times.

_T_ 18. Urine that has been standing at room temperature for a while may smell like ammonia.

_T_ 19. Blood for manual cell counts has to be diluted.

_F_ 20. Anything with a pH below 7 is alkaline.

Matching

   a. Hematocrit
   b. Urinalysis
   c. Erythrocyte sedimentation rate
   d. Red blood cell count
   e. White blood cell count
   f. Platelet count
   g. Differential count
   h. Bleeding time
   i. ABO slide typing
   j. Gram staining
   k. Occult blood

_b_ 21. Physical and chemical examination of urine

_k_ 22. Checking feces for hidden blood

_f_ 23. Count inside the entire center square of the hemacytometer

_a_ 24. Capillary tubes of blood have to be centrifuged

_i_ 25. Determines blood types

_c_ 26. Blood has to sit in a rack for 1 hour

_g_ 27. Counting percentage of each type of white blood cell

_j_ 28. Adding dye to a bacterial smear to identify types of bacteria

_h_ 29. Evaluates blood's clotting ability

_e_ 30. Count cells within four large corner squares

_d_ 31. Count only in four corner squares and middle square of large middle square

Answers

1. **False** Physical examination of urine consists of looking at color, and transparency, checking smell, and testing specific gravity.
2. **True**
3. **False** Specific gravity is expressed as the ratio of the weight of a certain amount of urine as compared to the same amount of water.
4. **False** Cholesterol crystals found in urine are abnormal.
5. **True**
6. **False** Hematocrit is found by multiplying hemoglobin by 3, or conversely, hemoglobin is found by taking one-third of hematocrit.
7. **True**
8. **True**
9. **True**
10. **True**
11. **False** A mordant causes dye to adhere to cell walls.
12. **False** Safranin dyes the cell walls pinkish red.
13. **False** The best urine specimen is the first urine voided in the morning.
14. **False** Capillary puncture is done on the finger, earlobe, or heel. The median cephalic vein is used for venipuncture.
15. **True**
16. **True**
17. **False** A laboratory jacket should be worn at all times, but _closed-toed_ shoes are necessary in the laboratory.
18. **True**
19. **True**
20. **False** pH below 7 is acid; pH above 7 is alkaline.
21. **b** Physical and chemical examination of the urine is called urinalysis.
22. **k** Checking feces for hidden blood is referred to as an occult blood test.

23. **f** When counting platelets, the entire center square of the hemacytometer is used to count platelets, counting left to right, then right to left, and counting only the platelets inside the area or touching the top and left edges.
24. **a** After two heparinized capillary tubes of blood are collected, they have to be placed in the centrifuge directly across from each other. After centrifuging, they may be read on a hematocrit reader, averaged and recorded.
25. **i** ABO slide typing helps determine whether the blood is type A, type B, type O, or type AB.
26. **c** When testing the erythrocyte sedimentation rate, collected blood has to stand in a rack for 1 hour before the speed at which red blood cells settle can be determined.
27. **g** Counting each type of white blood cell after identifying whether it is a neutrophil, an eosinophil, a basophil, a monocyte, or a lymphocyte is called the differential count.
28. **j** Gram staining helps identify bacteria because certain stains adhere to certain types of bacteria while other stains may be washed away. By staining with different types of stains, bacteria show up more clearly and can be identified more easily due to the type of dye that adheres to the cell walls.
29. **h** Tests for bleeding time show the amount of time it takes for blood from an incision to clot; and thus the blood's clotting ability.
30. **e** Manual white cell counting uses the four large corner squares to identify and count cells.
31. **d** Manual red blood cell counting uses only the four corner squares and the middle square within the larger middle square.

18

Medication Administration

CHAPTER OUTLINE

Common Drugs and Use
Administration Guidelines
Prescriptions

I. COMMON DRUGS AND USE
   A. Antihistamines
      1. _Seldane:_ terfenadine
         a. Nondrowsy antihistamine
         b. Use: rhinitis and allergies
         c. Adverse reactions: first antihistamine with significant lack of adverse reactions
         d. Route: oral
   B. Spasmolytics/bronchial smooth muscle relaxers
      1. _Theophylline_, _Slo-Phyllin_, _Theo-Dur:_ aminophylline
         a. Use: helps asthma and emphysema symptoms by relaxing bronchial spasms
         b. Adverse reactions: palpitations, tachycardia, and hypotension
         c. Route: oral
      2. _Proventil_, _Ventolin:_ albuterol
         a. Use: decreases bronchospasms and decreases asthma and emphysema symptoms
         b. Adverse reactions: tremor, palpitations, and tachycardia
         c. Route: oral or inhalation
      3. _Adrenalin Chloride Solution:_ epinephrine
         a. Use: decreases bronchospasms, decreases asthma and emphysema symptoms, is the drug of choice for severe allergic reactions (anaphylaxis), increases heart rate and output, and increases blood pressure
         b. Adverse reactions: tremor, palpitations, and tachycardia
         c. Route: IM, SC, parenteral, or inhalation
   C. Antianginals
      1. _Inderal:_ propranolol hydrochloride
         a. Use: decreases angina, arrythmias, and hypertension
         b. Adverse reactions: lethargy, bradycardia, and hypotension
         c. Route: oral
      2. _Cardizem:_ diltiazem hydrochloride
         a. Use: dilates coronary arteries, decreases angina, and is antihypertensive
         b. Adverse reactions: lethargy, arrythmias, bradycardia, hypotension, and photosensitivity
         c. Route: oral
      3. _Procardia:_ nifedipine
         a. Use: dilates coronary arteries and decreases angina
         b. Adverse reactions: hypotension, palpitations, and dizziness
         c. Route: oral
      4. _Nitrostat:_ nitroglycerine (NTG)
         a. Use: increases blood flow in coronary arteries, decreases angina, and decreases hypertension

b. Adverse reactions: headache, weakness, orthostatic hypotension, tachycardia, and palpitations

c. Route: oral or skin patch (Transderm-Nitro: nitroglycerine transdermal system)

5. *Calan:* verapamil

    a. Use: dilates coronary arteries, and decreases angina

    b. Adverse reactions: dizziness, hypotension, and bradycardia

    c. Route: oral

D. Antihypertensives/diuretics

1. *Tenormin:* atenolol

    a. Use: decreases hypertension

    b. Adverse reactions: lethargy, bradycardia, and hypotension

    c. Tip: check pulse prior to administration; if less than 60, do not administer

    d. Route: oral

2. *Capoten:* catopril

    a. Use: decreases severe hypertension

    b. Adverse reactions: leukocytopenia (decreased white blood cells), tachycardia, and hypotension

    c. Route: oral

3. *Lopressor:* metoprolol

    a. Use: decreases hypertension

    b. Adverse reactions: bradycardia, lethargy, and hypotension

    c. Route: oral

4. Maxzide, Dyazide: triamterene hydrochlorothiazide (HCTZ)

    a. Use: diuretic and decreases hypertension

    b. Good choice when trying to avoid depletion of potassium (K)

    c. Route: oral

5. *Vasotec:* enalapril maleate

    a. Use: diuretic and decreases hypertension

    b. Adverse reactions: palpitations, arrythmias, and hypotension

    c. Route: oral

6. *Diuril:* chlorothiazide

    a. Use: decreases edema and hypertension, and is a diuretic

    b. Adverse reactions: hypokalemia (decreased potassium) and decreased blood cell counts (*Tip:* Encourage a potassium-rich diet)

    c. Route: oral

7. *Lasix:* furosemide

    a. Use: diuretic; for edema

    b. Adverse reactions: agranulocytosis, orthostatic hypotension, and hypokalemia

    c. Route: oral or IM

E. Cardiac glycosides
   1. *Lanoxin:* digoxin
      a. Use: strengthens heart contraction, used for CHF (congestive heart failure)
      b. Adverse reactions: weakness, lethargy, dizziness, hypotension, arrythmias, and photophobia
      c. Route: oral
      d. *Tip:* check pulse before administration, if below 60, do not administer
F. Antifungals
   1. *Monistat:* miconazole
      a. Use: vaginal candidiasis (fungal infection)
      b. Adverse reactions: burning, stinging, and irritation
      c. Route: topical (cream, lotion, or suppository) or aerosol
   2. *Fulvicin:* griseofulvin ultramicrosize
      a. Use: ringworm and fungal infections
      b. Adverse reactions: headache, nausea, vomiting, and granulocytopenia
      c. Route: oral
   3. *Mycostatin:* nystatin
      a. Use: infections caused by *Candida*
      b. Adverse reactions: nausea and vomiting
      c. Other forms: "swish and swallow" for oral thrush
      d. Route: oral, lozenge, or topical (vaginal cream)
G. Antiinfectives
   1. Penicillins
      a. *Augmentin:* amoxicillin and potassium clavulanate
         • Use: urinary tract infections and upper respiratory infections
         • Adverse reactions: decreased blood cell count, nausea, vomiting, anaphylaxis, and superinfections due to overgrowth of nonsusceptible organisms
         • Route: oral or chewable
      b. *Amoxil:* moxicillin
         • Use: systemic infections and urinary tract infections
         • Adverse reactions: decreased blood cell count, nausea, vomiting, anaphylaxis, and superinfections
         • Route: oral or chewable
   2. Cephalosporins
      a. *Ceclor:* cefaclor
         • Use: urinary tract infections, upper respiratory infections, and otitis media
         • Adverse reactions: decreased blood cell count, nausea, vomiting, and superinfections
         • Route: oral

3. Fluoroquinolines
   a. *Cipro:* ciprofloxacin hydrochloride
      • Use: urinary tract infections and upper respiratory infections
      • Adverse reactions: decreased blood cell count and superinfections
      • Route: oral or ophthalmic solution
4. Mycin drugs
   a. *E-Mycin:* erythromycin base
      • Use: upper respiratory infections, urinary tract infections, and prophylaxis for dental procedures
      • Adverse reactions: nausea, vomiting, hearing loss, superinfections, and anaphylaxis
      • Route: oral, topical, or ophthalmic ointment
      • Usual drug of choice if patient is allergic to penicillin
5. Sulfonamides
   a. *Septra, Bactrim:* trimethoprim and sulfamethoxazole
      • Use: urinary tract infections, bronchitis, and otitis media
      • Adverse reactions: decreased blood cell count, nausea, vomiting, photosensitivity, anaphylaxis, and crystaluria
      • Route: oral
6. *Achromycin:* tetracycline
   a. Use: broad-spectrum antimicrobial
   b. Adverse reactions: nausea, vomiting, diarrhea, photosensitivity, and discoloration of nails and teeth
   c. Warnings: not to be given to children below age 8 (or pregnant women), due to tooth discoloration; do not take with dairy products or antacids
   d. Route: oral, topical, IM, or ophthalmic
H. Gastrointestinal drugs
   1. *Zantac:* ranitidine hydrochloride
      a. Use: decreases ulcers and decreases gastric acid secretions
      b. Adverse reactions: decreased blood cell count, headache, nausea, and constipation
      c. Route: oral or IM
   2. *Carafate:* sucralfate
      a. Use: decreases ulcers
      b. Adverse reactions: nausea and constipation
      c. Route: oral
   3. *Tagamet:* cimetidine
      a. Use: decreases ulcers
      b. Adverse reactions: decreased blood cell count, headache, and diarrhea
      c. Route: oral or IM

I. Sedatives/hypnotics
   1. *Halcion:* triazolam
      a. Use: decreases insomnia
      b. Adverse reactions: headache, nausea, vomiting, and rebound insomnia
      c. Schedule IV drug
      d. Route: oral
   2. *Dalmane:* flurazepam hydrochloride
      a. Use: decreases insomnia
      b. Adverse reactions: decreased blood cell count, lethargy, and headache
      c. Schedule IV drug
      d. Route: oral
   3. *Noctec:* chloral hydrate
      a. Use: decreases insomnia
      b. Adverse reactions: decreased blood cell count, nausea, vomiting, and drowsiness
      c. Schedule IV drug
      d. Route: oral or suppository
J. Antiinflammatory nonsteroidal drugs
   1. *Feldene:* piroxicam
      a. Use: analgesic (decreases pain), decreases inflammation, and is antipyretic (reduces fever)
      b. Adverse reactions: increased bleeding, GI problems, photosensitivity, and anemia
      c. Route: oral
   2. *Motrin, Advil:* ibuprofen
      a. Use: reduces inflammation, analgesic, antipyretic, and antiarthritic
      b. Adverse reactions: increased bleeding and tinnitus
      c. Route: oral
   3. *Naprosyn, Anaprox:* naproxen
      a. Use: antiarthritic and analgesic
      b. Adverse reactions: increased bleeding and headache
      c. Route: oral
   4. *Voltaren:* diclofenac sodium
      a. Use: antiarthritic and after cataract surgery is used to decrease inflammation
      b. Adverse reactions: nausea, vomiting; and stinging in the eyes and increased eye pressure
      c. Route: oral or ophthalmic
K. Muscle relaxers
   1. *Robaxin:* methocarbamol
      a. Use: decreases pain in acute musculoskeletal conditions
      b. Adverse reactions: headache, hypotension, nausea, GI problems, and anaphylaxis
      c. Route: oral or IM

2. *Flexeril:* cyclobenzaprine hydrochloride
   a. Use: decreases pain and decreases muscle spasms
   b. Adverse reactions: drowsiness, tachycardia, and dizziness
   c. Route: oral
L. Antianxiety agents
   1. *Valium:* diazepam
      a. Use: decreases tension, muscle spasms, and seizures
      b. Adverse reactions: lethargy, bradycardia, hypotension, and decreased respirations
      c. Schedule IV drug
      d. Route: oral or IM
   2. *Xanax:* alprazolam
      a. Use: decreases anxiety and tension
      b. Adverse reactions: drowsiness, hypotension, nausea, and vomiting
      c. Schedule IV drug
      d. Route: oral
M. Hormones/replacements
   1. *Premarin:* estrogen
      a. Use: abnormal uterine bleeding, prostate and breast cancer, and osteoporosis
      b. Adverse reactions: dizziness, increased risk of stroke or MI, nausea, vomiting, and weight changes
      c. Route: oral, IM, or vaginal cream
   2. *Lo-Ovral:* estrogen with progesterone
      a. Use: oral contraceptive
      b. Adverse reactions: headache, dizziness, thromboemboli, hypertension, nausea, and vomiting
      c. Route: oral
   3. *Triphasil:* estradiol and levonorgestrel
      a. Use: oral contraceptive
      b. Adverse reactions: headache, thromboemboli, and hypertension
      c. Route: oral
   4. *Provera:* medroxyprogesterone acetate
      a. Use: supresses ovulation, for abnormal bleeding, amenorrhea, and endometrial cancer
      b. Adverse reactions: dizziness, lethargy, nausea, and vomiting
      c. Route: oral or IM
   5. *Synthroid:* levothyroxine sodium
      a. Use: thyroid hormone replacement, stimulates metabolism, for cretinism, and myxedema
      b. Adverse reactions: nervousness, tremor, tachycardia, palpitations, and arrythmias
      c. Route: oral or IM

6. *Mephyton:* phytonadione (vitamin K)
   a. Use: increases prothrombin needed for clotting
   b. Adverse reactions: dizziness, hypotension, nausea, vomiting, anaphylaxis, and cardiac irregularities
   c. Route: oral, IM, or SC
7. *Micro-K, Slow-K:* potassium chloride
   a. Use: replaces potassium
   b. Adverse reactions: hyperkalemia, hypotension, arrythmias, confusion, nausea, and vomiting
   c. Route: oral
8. *Feosol:* ferrous sulfate (category-hematinic)
   a. Use: iron replacement and anemia
   b. Adverse reactions: nausea, vomiting, constipation, and black stools
   c. Route: oral

N. Antihyperlipidemic
   1. *Mevacor:* lovastatin
      a. Use: lowers cholesterol
      b. Adverse reactions: flatus, nausea, and lens changes in the eyes
      c. Route: oral

O. Antidiabetics/hypoglycemics
   1. *Micronase:* glyburide
      a. Use: increases insulin release for type II (non-insulin dependent) diabetes
      b. Adverse reactions: bone marrow aplasia, nausea, and hypoglycemia
      c. Route: oral

P. Antiglaucoma ophthalmic drops
   1. *Timoptic:* timolol maleate
      a. Use: decreases pressure in the eyes
      b. Adverse reactions: CHF (congestive heart failure), bradycardia, and headache
      c. Route: oral or ophthalmic

Q. Antiacnes
   1. *Retin-A:* tretinoin
      a. Use: decreases acne
      b. Adverse reactions: blistered skin and photosensitivity where used
      c. Route: topical only

R. Nonnarcotic analgesics
   1. *Darvocet-N:* acetaminophen and propoxyphene napsylate
      a. Use: mild to moderate pain
      b. Adverse reaction: dizziness, headache, and euphoria
      c. Schedule IV drug
      d. Route: oral

S. Anticoagulants
  1. *Coumadin:* warfarin sodium
     a. Use: decreases vitamin K to decrease clotting, treatment for pulmonary emboli and MI
     b. Adverse reactions: hemorrhage, nausea, vomiting, alopecia, and decreased white blood cell count
     c. Route: oral or IM
T. Antidepressants
  1. *Prozac:* fluoxetine hydrochloride
     a. Use: decreases depression
     b. Adverse reactions: headache, nervousness, nausea, and vomiting
     c. Route: oral
U. Immunizations
  1. *DTP* (diptheria, tetanus, pertussis): give at 2, 4, 6, and 18 months, and at 5 years; tetanus and diptheria every 10 years thereafter
  2. *OPV* (oral polio vaccine): give at 2, 4, and 18 months, and at 4 to 6 years
  3. *MMR* [measles (i.e., rubeola); mumps; rubella (i.e., German measles)]: give at 12 months, and 5 years
  4. *Haemophilus influenza:* give at 2, 4, 6, and 15 months
  5. New combination childhood vaccine (Tetramune): give at 2, 4, 6, and 15 months for diptheria, tetanus, pertussis (whooping cough), and *Haemophilus influenzae* type B (the leading cause of meningitis)

II. ADMINISTRATION GUIDELINES
  A. "Eight rights of giving medicine" (right patient, right drug, right dose, right route, right time, right documentation, right technique, right follow-up)
     1. Right patient
        a. Identification of the patient without a doubt
     2. Right drug
        a. Label is read three times
           • When removing medicine from the shelf
           • When pouring the medicine
           • When returning the medicine to the shelf prior to giving it to the patient
        b. Check the medicine against the doctor's order
        c. Verify the medicine when writing is not clear or spelling of the drug name is similar to that of another drug
        d. Ingredients may be the same but the names differ
           • *Generic:* not sold under a specific trade name
           • *Official:* name is listed in the USP/NF (United States Pharmacopeia/National Formulary), the official list of standard drugs
           • *Trade name:* brand name given the same drug made made by different companies

3. Right dose
   a. Check the package insert
   b. Use the PDR *(Physicians' Desk Reference)* or other drug reference books to check dosage
   c. Check dosage measured against the dosage ordered
   d. Calculations of dosage
      - Knowledge of apothecary and metric system
      - General formula:

$$\text{dosage} = \frac{\text{doctor's order}}{\text{Strength of medicine you have on hand}}$$

   Example: Doctor orders 250 mg; you have 50-mg tablets.

$$\frac{250 \text{mg}}{50 \text{ mg / tablet}} = 5 \text{ tablets}$$

      - Children's dosage:

$$\text{dosage} = \text{patient age} \ \times \ \frac{\text{usual adult dose}}{150 \text{ months (adult age)}}$$

   Example: $10 \text{ months} \ \times \ \dfrac{300 \text{ mg}}{150 \text{ months}} \ = \ 20 \text{ mg}$

$$\text{dosage} = \text{patient weight} \ \times \ \frac{\text{usual adult dose}}{150 \text{ pounds (adult weight)}}$$

   Example: $50 \text{ lbs} \ \times \ \dfrac{300 \text{ mg}}{150 \text{ lbs}} \ = \ 100 \text{ mg}$

4. Right route
   a. *Oral* (abbreviation—P.O.): by mouth
      - Safest but slowest route
      - Liquid, tablets, and capsules
      - Absorption is through the stomach and intestines (check if medicine should be taken on a full or empty stomach, with dairy products, etc.)
      - Timed-release capsules or enteric-coated tabs (do not crush)
      - If tablets are not scored, do not halve
   b. *Buccal (abbreviation—buc.):* inside the cheek
      - Absorption is through mucous membranes (do not chew or swallow)
   c. *Topical* (directions will state how to apply)
      - Absorption is slow
      - Lotions are patted on; drops (gtt.) are for eyes or ears; sprays; bladder, wound, or vaginal irrigations

d. _Rectal and vaginal_ (p.r. or R. = rectal; p.v. = vaginal)
- Absorption is slow and irregular
- Cream, suppository, ointment (ung.), foam (ensure that patients receive instructions on how to administer so that they don't swallow suppositories)
- Rectal: for vomiting patient who cannot keep medications down
- Effects: may be local

e. _Inhalation:_ breathe in the medication
- Sprays, mist, steam, and puffs
- Use care in cleaning equipment

f. _Transdermal_ (patch)
- Absorption is slow
- Systemic effects

g. _Sublingual_ (under the tongue)
- Absorption is through mucous membranes
- Systemic effects
Example: Nitroglycerine tablets used in angina to dilate coronary arteries to increase oxygen to the heart muscle.

h. _Parenteral_ (injecting with needle and syringe)
- Absorption is rapid
- Intramuscular
- Intradermal
- Subcutaneous
- Intravenous (not done by medical assistants)

5. Right time
   a. Maximum effectiveness: drugs given at the correct time with the correct intervals of time between dosages.

6. Right documentation
   a. Exact process of giving medication is written in the patient's chart including drug, dose, route, time, and so on

7. Right technique
   a. Technique is correct

8. Right follow-up
   a. Assess the patient for untoward reactions and allergies; note whether patient experienced pain decrease after taking pain medication; note changes in vital signs after medication administration, and so on
   b. Documentation in the patient's chart of follow-up
   Example: Vital signs taken; pulse 70 (after cardiac drugs)
   Example: Patient observed for 20 minutes with no signs of allergic or untoward reactions (after possibility of reaction to injection)

B. Parenteral medication administration

1. Equipment
   a. _Syringes:_ must be sterile inside
   - Standard volume is 0 to 3 ml (cc)

- Insulin is given in units (standard volume of syringe: 100 units)
- Tuberculin or allergy syringes: for small dosages; calibrated in hundredths of a cubic centimeter

b. *Needles:* must be sterile and without burrs
- *Gauges:* 18 to 21 for viscous medications; 22 to 26 for thinner, more liquid medications
- *Lengths:* $\frac{3}{8}$ to $\frac{5}{8}$-inch for intradermal and subcutaneous; 1 to 1-$\frac{1}{2}$ inches for intramuscular

c. *Ampules of medication:* glass containers with bulb that will be broken or filed off for aspiration of medication

d. *Vials of medication:* containers with rubber stoppers (must be cleansed with alcohol prior to aspiration of medication)

2. Intradermal injections
a. *Sites:* into the upper layers of skin of the forearm or the back

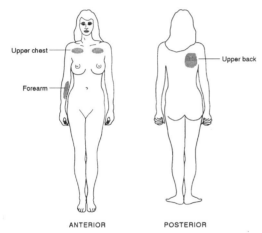

Figure 18-1 Intradermal injection sites.

b. *Use:* allergy testing and TB testing
c. *Amounts:* no more than 0.3 cc given
d. *Needle size:* $\frac{3}{8}$ to $\frac{5}{8}$ inch; 26 to 27 gauge
e. *Angle:* almost parallel to skin (10 to 15 degrees); will form a bleb when injected

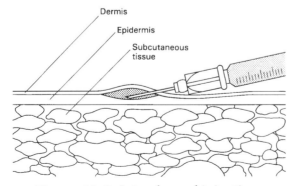

Figure 18-2 Intradermal injection.

     f. No aspiration needed prior to injection

     g. Tine tests pressed 1 to 2 mm in depth and held a second or two

  3. Subcutaneous injections

     a. *Sites:* within fatty layers of skin on the upper arm, thigh, or abdomen

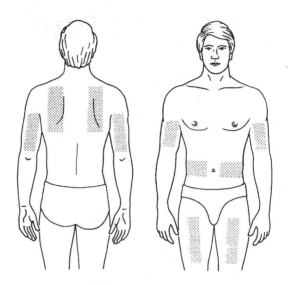

Figure 18-3 Subcutaneous injection sites.

     b. *Use:* insulin, local anesthesia, epinephrine, and heparin

     c. *Amounts:* 0.1 to 2 ml (cc)

     d. *Needle size:* $\frac{1}{2}$ to $\frac{5}{8}$-inch; 24 to 28 gauge

     e. *Angle:* 45 degrees (sometimes insulin is given at a 90-degree angle)

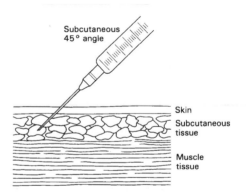

Figure 18-4 Subcutaneous injection.

     f. Aspiration is needed prior to injection (except insulin or heparin) to be sure that injection is not intravenous

4. Intramuscular injections
   a. *Sites:* within a muscle

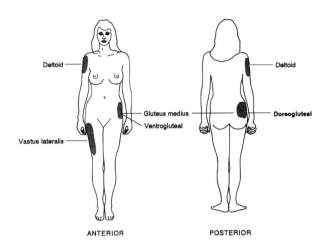

Figure 18-5 Intramuscular injection sites.

- Deltoid muscle: upper arm, halfway between the top of the shoulder (acromion) and the armpit; the amount is 0 to 2 ml (cc)
- Vastus lateralis muscle: midlateral thigh; the amount is 0 to 5 ml (cc); this is the safest parenteral route for infants and children
- Ventrogluteal site (gluteus medius muscle): on right side of the patient, place left palm of the hand on the greater trochanter and the index finger on the anterior, superior iliac spine; spread the middle finger apart and inject into the "V" that is made by the index and middle fingers; the amount is 0 to 5 ml (cc).
- Dorsogluteal site (gluteus medius muscle): inject above an imaginary line from the posterior iliac spine to the greater trochanter of the femur; the amount is 0 to 5 ml (cc)

   b. *Use:* penicillin and corticosteroid drugs
   c. *Amounts:* 0 to 5 ml (cc); see individual sites for amounts
   d. *Needle size:* 1 to 1-1/2-inches; 18 to 23 gauge
   e. *Angle:* usually 90 degrees

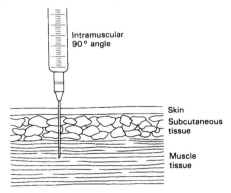

Figure 18-6 Intramuscular injection.

f. Aspiration is advised to be certain that needle is not in a vein or an artery

g. Avoid major nerves and vessels by location of correct injection site (especially avoid the sciatic nerve in the buttocks area)

5. Technique

a. Sterile technique is used: wipe area to be injected with a circular motion, inside out; use a sterile needle, sterile medication, and sterile area of syringe touching the medication (hands are always washed; Universal Precautions are always used)

b. Eight rights are used (right patient, right drug, right dose, right time, right route, right documentation, right technique, and right follow-up)

c. Medication is compared with doctor's orders and checked three times to ensure that the correct drug is being used

d. Inspect the needle for burrs; inspect the medication for quality and expiration date

e. Wipe vial with antiseptic; air equal to the amount of medicine to be withdrawn is injected into the vial and the medicine withdrawn

f. *Ampule:* break and withdraw medicine (not necessary to inject air since no equalization of pressure is needed with an ampule)

g. Bubbles in a syringe are removed by gently tapping and pushing plunger to eliminate (recheck to be sure of correct dosage)

h. Needle is inserted quickly and at the correct angle: for subcutaneous injections, pinch up the skin; for intradermal and intramuscular, pull the skin area taut

i. *Aspiration:* to ensure a needle is not in a vein or an artery, pull back gently on plunger to see if blood is aspirated (no aspiration needed for intradermal; no aspiration needed for insulin or heparin injected subcutaneously)

j. Medication is injected slowly, the needle is removed quickly, and pressure is applied with sterile gauze at the site

k. Needle and syringe are deposited as a unit in a puncture-proof container (no recapping is necessary to avoid possible needle stick)

l. Process is entered on the patient's chart, including documentation of eight rights.

Example: Patient: Jenny Hemby   12-12-94
2:15 pm 50 mg. Demerol IM right ventrogluteal area for pain ordered per J. Langston, MD.
Tolerated well. Vital signs monitored before and after
P-70, R-16, B/P-120/90 Patient states, "pain eased".

m. Observation of patient is necessary if there is a possibility of an allergic reaction or a change in vital signs

C. Prescriptions

1. *Date:* cannot be filled after a certain amount of time
2. *Patient data:* name and address
3. *Superscription:* Rx means "take"
4. *Inscription:* drug, dosage, and form
5. *Subscription:* amount to be dispensed
6. *Signature:* "Sig" means "write on label" the instructions to the patient (whether to take with food or on an empty stomach, how often to take, whether refrigeration is needed, and so on)
7. *Refills:* indicate whether or not to be refilled and how many times
8. *Physician's signature:* doctor must sign name and title
9. DEA number is usually imprinted on all prescriptions
10. Special DEA forms are needed for office prescriptions if controlled substances are to be administered in the doctor's office
11. Warning: keep prescription forms locked up
12. *Verbal orders:* be sure to record drug given and other pertinent information, but always get the doctor's signature showing that he/she ordered the drug. Check accuracy of the verbal order by repeating dosage, drug, and so on, to the physician.

QUESTIONS

Match the category of drug and the drug.
- a. Antidepressant
- b. Anticoagulant
- c. Antiacne
- d. Antidiabetic/hypoglycemic
- e. Antihyperlipidemic

_d_ 1. Micronase
_e_ 2. Mevacor
_b_ 3. Coumadin
_a_ 4. Prozac
_c_ 5. Retin-A

- a. Antiglaucoma
- b. Hematinic
- c. Oral contraceptive
- d. Thyroid replacement
- e. Antianxiety

_c_ 6. Triphasil
_a_ 7. Timoptic
_b_ 8. Feosol
_e_ 9. Valium
_d_ 10. Synthroid

- a. Muscle relaxant
- b. Antiinflammatory
- c. Antiinflammatory ophthalmic drops after cataract surgery
- d. Sedative
- e. GI drug to decrease ulcers

_b_ 11. Feldene
_e_ 12. Carafate
_a_ 13. Robaxin
_d_ 14. Halcion
_c_ 15. Voltaren

- a. Antiinfective
- b. Antifungal against _Candida_
- c. Cardiac glycoside
- d. Diuretic
- e. Antihistamine

_c_ 16. Lanoxin
_a_ 17. penicillins
_e_ 18. Seldane (nondrowsy)
_d_ 19. Lasix
_b_ 20. Mycostatin

- a. Antihypertensive
- b. Smooth muscle relaxant to decrease bronchial spasms
- c. Antianginal
- d. Diuretic
- e. Antiinfective

_e_ 21. cephalosporins
_b_ 22. Proventil, Ventolin
_d_ 23. Diuril
_a_ 24. Tenormin
_c_ 25. Nitrostat

True-False

_T_ 26. You must read the label of a drug three times before administering it to a patient: once when removing it from the shelf, once before pouring it, and once before you replace it back on the shelf prior to giving it to the patient.

_F_ 27. The right dose of a drug for an adult will be the right dose for a child.

_T_ 28. If the doctor orders 500 mg of a parenteral medication and the label indicates 250 mg/ml, the correct amount to be given is 2 ml.

_F_ 29. The safest route to give medications is intravenous.

_F_ 30. Absorption of medication through the mucous membranes of the cheek is the sublingual route.

I 31. Topical medication is used for local effects.

T 32. A rectal suppository or a parenteral injection may be necessary when a patient is vomiting.

33. List the eight rights of giving medications.

34. List the three types of parenteral injections a medical assistant can give,

explain the sites used, the usual amounts given, the needle size, the angle usually used, and whether or not aspiration is necessary.

35. Give an example of medication for each type of parenteral injection.

36. List the parts of a prescription and explain each part.

Answers

1. d Micronase is an antidiabetic.
2. e Mevacor is an antihyperlipidemic.
3. b Coumadin is an anticoagulant.
4. a Prozac is an antidepressant.
5. c Retin-A is an antiacne medication.
6. c Triphasil is an oral contraceptive.
7. a Timoptic is an antiglaucoma medication.
8. b Feosol is a hematinic or iron replacement.
9. e Valium is an antianxiety medication.
10. d Synthroid is a thyroid replacement.
11. b Feldene is an antiinflammatory.
12. e Carafate is a gastrointestinal (GI) medication used to decrease ulcers.
13. a Robaxin is a muscle relaxant.
14. d Halcion is a sedative.
15. c Voltaren is used after cataract surgery to decrease inflammation.
16. c Lanoxin is a cardiac glycoside that makes the heart a more effective pump.
17. a Penicillins are antiinfectives.
18. e Seldane is a nondrowsy antihistamine.
19. d Lasix is a diuretic.
20. b Mycostatin is an antifungal against *Candida*.
21. e Cephalosporins are broad-spectrum antiinfectives.
22. b Proventil and Ventolin are smooth muscle relaxants that reduce bronchospasms.
23. d Diuril is a diuretic.
24. a Tenormin is an antihypertensive.
25. c Nitrostat is an antianginal.
26. True Before giving any patient a medication, you must read the label three times: once when you remove the medication from the shelf, once when you pour the medication, and once when you put the medication back on the shelf, prior to giving it to the patient.
27. False Children's doses will be different from adult doses unless the child is the size or

weight of an adult or at least 12-$\frac{1}{2}$ years of age. When giving medications to children, you may use the standard formulas for calculating children's doses.

28. True The formula for calculating medication is want/have or

$$\frac{\text{what the doctor orders}}{\text{what you have}}$$

Therefore, 500 mg divided by 250 mg/ml = 2 ml

29. False The safest route is the oral route.
30. False Buccal medication is absorbed in the mucous membranes of the cheek. Sublingual medication is absorbed under the tongue.
31. True Topical medication is administered for the local effects. It is used on the problem area.
32. True The rectal route or an injection is indicated when a patient is vomiting and cannot keep a medication down.
33. The eight rights of administering a medication are: 1. the right patient; 2. the right drug; 3. the right dose; 4. the right route; 5. the right time; 6. the right documentation; 7. the right technique; 8. the right follow-up.
34. The three categories of parenteral medication a medical assistant can give and explanations of each are as follows:
Intradermal: sites: lower arm and back—upper layer of skin; needle: $\frac{3}{8}$ to $\frac{5}{8}$-inch; 26 to 27 gauge; amount: up to 0.3 cc; angle: almost parallel to skin, 10 to 15 degrees; no aspiration is needed.
Subcutaneous: sites: arm, thigh, and abdomen—fatty layer of skin; needle: $\frac{1}{2}$ to $\frac{5}{8}$- inch; 24 to 28 gauge; amount: 0.1 to 2 cc; angle: 45 degrees; aspirate except with insulin and heparin.

Intramuscular: sites: deltoid, vastus lateralis, dorsogluteal, ventrogluteal deep in the muscle mass; needle: 1 to 1-½-inches; 18 to 23 gauge; amount: 0 to 5 cc; angle : 90 degrees; aspiration is necessary to be sure the needle is not in a vein or an artery.

35.   Examples of medications given in each category of parenteral medication are:
Intradermal: TB test and allergy tests
Subcutaneous: heparin and insulin
Intramuscular: penicillin

36.   The parts of a prescription are as follows: date, name, and address of the patient; superscription or Rx; inscription includes the name of the drug, the dose, form, and amount; subscription tells the amount to dispense; signature indicates what directions to write on the label; refills; and doctor's signature. The DEA number should appear on the prescription as well.

19

Emergencies and First Aid

CHAPTER OUTLINE

Guides for Emergencies
Cardiopulmonary Resuscitation
Types of Emergencies and Treatments

I. GUIDES FOR EMERGENCIES
   A. *Scope of practice:* only administer treatment within limitations of profession and standard office protocol
   B. Listing of emergency numbers should be convenient: 911 and poison control centers
   C. Preventive measures should be practiced and taught to patients
   D. Crash cart or tray should be on hand
      1. Expiration dates should be checked regularly and documented
      2. Inventory and restocking should be done after all emergencies
      3. Drills should be practiced and roles assigned
      4. Batteries should be checked and replaced as needed in battery-operated equipment; keep spares on hand
   E. Emergency exits should be marked appropriately, fire extinguishers updated, and other emergency supplies and equipment marked and updated as needed; office staff must be aware of emergency procedures, locations, and equipment

II. CARDIOPULMONARY RESUSCITATION (CPR)
Always check for your own safety by inspecting the scene for hazards; use a mask or barrier between you and the victim.
   A. *Responsiveness of patient:* Ask, "Are you OK?"
   B. *ABCs of CPR*
      1. *A = Airway:* Is the airway open? Can the head be repositioned to open the airway? Avoid moving the head, however, if a neck injury is possible.
      2. *B = Breathing*
         a. Look: Is the chest moving up and down?
         b. Listen: With ear over patient's mouth, do you hear breathing?
         c. Feel: With ear over patient's mouth and hand on chest, do you feel air or chest movement?
      3. *C = Circulation:* When you feel the patient's carotid artery (beside the Adam's apple), is there a pulse?
   C. *No breathing, but has pulse:* rescue breaths are needed
      1. *Adult:* one breath every 5 seconds
      2. *Child:* one breath every 3 seconds
      3. *Infant:* one breath every 3 seconds
   D. *No breathing, no pulse:* must initiate CPR, breathing for the patient and performing chest compressions
      1. *Breathing:* adult and child—hold the patient's nose and blow breaths into the mouth (if using a mask, it will fit over the mouth and nose). infant—rescuer's mouth over infant's mouth and nose

2. *Chest compressions*
   a. Site
      - *Adult and child:* two finger widths above sternal notch or ziphoid process
      - *Infant:* place index finger sideways between nipples over sternal area, place middle and ring fingers next to index finger, lift index finger, and other two fingers are in place
   b. *Adult:* use both hands, one over the other (with heel of hand on sternum, fingertips up)
   c. *Child (8 years old and below, but not an infant):* use heel of one hand
   d. *Infant:* use two fingers only
   e. *Count:* one-person CPR
      - *Adult:* 15 compressions per two breaths for 4 cycles; then reevaluate need for CPR, continuing if necessary (rate = 80 to 100 times per minute)
      - *Child:* 5 compressions per one breath for 20 cycles; then reevaluate need for CPR, continuing if necessary (rate = 100 times per minute)
      - *Infant:* 5 compressions per one puff of breath for 20 cycles, continuing CPR after reevaluation of no pulse or breaths (rate = at least 100 times per minute); brachial pulse checked instead of carotid pulse
   f. Two-person CPR
      - *Adult:* breaths by one rescuer, compressions by the other; compressor calls for switch when tired
      - 5 compressions per one breath for 20 cycles, continuing CPR after reevaluation of no pulse or breaths (rate = 80 to 100 times per minute for compressions)

III. TYPES OF EMERGENCIES AND TREATMENTS

A. *Choking:* use Heimlich maneuver

1. Adult and child
   a. *Coughing and speaking:* leave patient alone; patient may be able to recover without help
   b. *Universal sign:* clutching throat (shows need for help); from behind the patient, put arms around (like a bear hug), and with one hand covering balled-up fist, swiftly give upward thrust below the ribs and above the umbilicus
   c. Upward thrusts are continued until patient coughs out foreign matter or until the patient becomes unconscious
   d. *Unconscious patient:* straddle and continue upward thrusts up to five times between the umbilicus and toward the rib cage using hand-over-hand method with heel of hand
   e. *No change:* if nothing is coughed out, insert hooked finger in back of throat (finger sweep) and try to expel the object from an adult (for a child you must inspect the mouth and do finger sweep only if an object is seen)

        f. Upward thrusts and finger sweeps are continued until the object is out or help arrives

        g. CPR is initiated, if needed, after the object is expelled

    2. Infant

        a. Five back blows between shoulder blades with head of infant downward, then five chest compressions (same placement as CPR)

        b. Back blows and chest compressions are continued until object is expelled

        c. Mouth is checked after back blows and compressions to see if the object can be finger-swept out of the mouth

        d. CPR is initiated, if needed, after the object is expelled

B. *Heart attack* (MI—myocardial infarction)

    1. *Symptoms:* pressure, squeezing sensation in the chest behind the sternum; pain may radiate to neck or shoulder, the patient may be extremely anxious, sweating, pale, and may have mild indigestion-like sensation; the patient may deny symptoms

    2. Complete rest is needed; nitroglycerine is given (if patient has it), 911 is called, CPR is initiated if needed, and an EKG is usually done

C. *Stroke* (CVA—cerebrovascular accident)

    1. *Symptoms:* confusion, slurred speech, dizziness, weakness or paralysis on one side of body, and unequal pupils

    2. Allow complete rest, maintain the airway, place on side if secretions are draining, and call 911

D. *Burns*

    1. *First degree:* first layer of skin has redness but no blistering

        a. Immerse in cool water or cover with a sterile wet compress

    2. *Second degree:* deeper burn than first degree with redness and blistering

        a. Immerse in cool water 1 to 2 hours and cover with a dry sterile dressing

    3. *Third degree:* deeper layers and may include muscle tissue; nerve endings may be destroyed

        a. Cover with thick sterile dressing; if clothing is burned into and adhering to the skin; do not try to remove

        b. Infection is a risk; may need antibiotics

        c. Dehydration is a risk; may need IV fluids

    4. *Chemical burns:* rinse copiously and cover with a sterile dressing (if burn agent is a powdered chemical, try to brush it off first)

    5. Debridement may be necessary as the area heals and dead tissue sloughs off

E. *Bleeding*

    1. Direct pressure with sterile compress

a. Use additional pads if necessary, but do not replace the old pad with a new one because you will disturb the clotting process
2. Elevate injured part (if possible)
3. *Pressure points:* apply pressure on the pressure point between the bleeder and the heart if direct pressure or elevation does not help

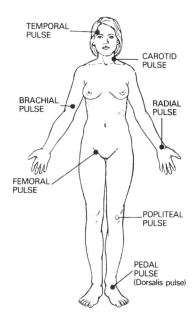

Figure 19-2 Pressure points of the body.

a. *Common carotid:* above the clavicle, press backward
b. *Temporal:* side of the face in front of the ear
c. *Subclavian:* behind the clavicle toward the first rib
d. *Axillary:* underarm area
e. *Brachial:* above the bend of the elbow
f. *Radial:* thumb side of the wrist
g. *Abdominal:* press against the lumbar vertebrae toward the left
h. *Femoral:* press against the groin area with leg abducted and rotated outward
i. *Popliteal:* back of the knee
4. *Tourniquet:* use only as a last resort—always note the time tourniquet was applied (usually on patient's forehead), and use only as life or death measure
5. *Shock:* may occur with severe bleeding, internally or externally; monitor blood pressure
F. *Shock:* extremely low blood pressure
1. *Symptoms:* pale, clammy skin; weak, rapid pulse; low blood pressure; dyspnea; and weakness

2. _Treatment:_ Use Trendelenburg position (legs elevated unless patient has a head or chest injury or dyspnea); maintain airway and continually check vital signs; keep NPO (nothing by mouth) and call 911

    a. _Traumatic shock:_ fluids lost outside the cells, as in large burned areas

    b. _Hypovolemic or hemorrhagic shock:_ internal or external blood loss; decrease in blood volume

    c. _Cardiogenic shock:_ decrease of the heart's ability to pump

    d. _Septic shock:_ severe bacterial infection

    e. _Neurogenic shock:_ fainting, tone of vessels decreased and dilated; thus a drop in blood pressure and heart rate

    f. _Anaphylactic shock:_ life-threatening allergic or sensitivity reaction to the extreme; edema, decreased blood pressure, dyspnea, and tachycardia

G. _Poisoning_

1. _Symptoms:_ burns around the mouth, nausea, cramps, shallow breathing, loss of consciousness, and convulsions
2. Dilute poison by drinking liquids (water or milk)
3. Syrup of ipecac to induce vomiting unless contraindicated (as with corrosives and caustics); induce only if patient is conscious
4. Vomitus and container of poison should be carried to the hospital with the patient
5. Activated charcoal is administered after vomiting to absorb residual poison

H. _Convulsions_

1. _Symptoms:_ jerking, spasmodic movements of a part or of the entire body
2. _Treatment:_ protect the head, maintain the airway, and nothing by mouth; after seizure, position on the side to promote drainage and prevent choking; call 911 if necessary

I. *Fractures*

   1. Types

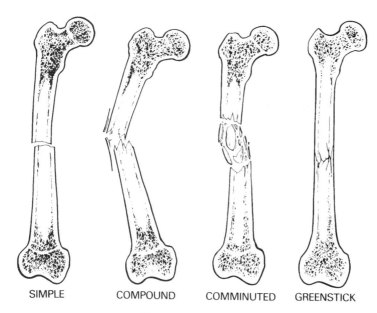

SIMPLE   COMPOUND   COMMINUTED   GREENSTICK

Figure 19-2 Different types of bone fractures.

     a. *Simple:* no open wound
     b. *Compound:* open wound
     c. *Comminuted:* broken into more than two pieces
     d. *Greenstick:* part of the bone split away like a green stick
     e. *Transverse:* break across the bone
     f. *Oblique:* break slants across the bone
     g. *Spiral:* break spirals around the bone
     h. *Impacted:* part of the bone is compressed into another part
     i. *Depressed:* bone is driven inward

   2. *Treatment:* restraint to prevent movement, elevation (if possible), mild compression, splinting, and ice pack; x-ray is usually done and doctor may perform reduction of the fracture

J. *Asthmatic attacks*

   1. *Symptoms:* shortness of breath, choking, and wheezing
   2. *Treatment:* medicate with bronchodilators, inhalation therapy, and mucolytics
   3. Avoid excessive exercise, laughing, coughing, and stress

K. *Insect stings*

   1. *Symptoms:* edema, itching, pain, and anaphylaxis (shock = low blood pressure, dyspnea, and edema of the airways)
   2. *Treatment:* remove stinger without squeezing, apply ice, give antihistamines for itching and anaphylaxis, and give epinephrine if needed for full-blown anaphylactic shock

L. *Diabetic coma/hyperglycemia*

    1. *Symptoms:* dry, flushed skin; drowsiness, vomiting, air hunger, fruity breath smell, and intense thirst

    2. *Treatment:* increased insulin (however, if not sure if diabetic coma or insulin shock, best to give sugar because insulin shock without treatment can have dire consequences)

    3. *Cause:* too little insulin, too much sugar, or stress

M. *Insulin shock/hypoglycemia*

    1. *Symptoms:* moist, pale skin; excitement, shallow or normal respirations, and bounding pulse

    2. *Treatment:* give food containing sugar

    3. *Cause:* too much insulin, not enough to eat, or increased exercise

N. *Foreign body in the eye or ear*

    1. Irrigate as necessary to remove the object; if instrumentation is necessary, a doctor should perform the procedure

O. *Syncope* (fainting)

    1. Loosen clothing and position the patient so that the head is below the heart

1. Name three general guides for emergencies.

2. List and explain the ABCs of CPR.

3. What are the rates for rescue breaths?

4. What are the rates of breathing and chest compressions in one-person CPR?

5. What is the hand placement for an adult, child, and infant in CPR?

6. Explain the treatment for a conscious choking adult and child.

7. Explain the treatment for a choking infant.

8. Explain the treatment for an unconscious choking adult and child.

9. Could a patient have a heart attack without realizing it?

10. Which degree of burn has no blistering?

11. Describe four measures to take when a patient is bleeding.

12. A victim of shock will have (high/low) blood pressure.

13. What is the first step to take in all poisonings?

14. A fracture with the bone piercing the skin is a (simple/compound) fracture.

15. Squeezing the stinger (is/is not) indicated as a treatment for insect bites?

16. Dry flushed skin is an indication of (diabetic coma/insulin shock).

17. Syncope is another term for ____.

Answers

1. General guides for emergencies are to stay calm, provide treatment within your legal scope of practice, practice and teach prevention, keep up-to-date and well-stocked crash carts, practice drills, and assign roles for emergencies.

2. A = Airway: Check to see if the patient's airway is open. Reposition the head if necessary.
   B = Breathing: Look, listen, and feel to see if the patient is breathing. If not, begin rescue breaths.
   C = Circulation: Check the carotid artery (beside the Adam's apple) for the adult and child, and the brachial artery (bend of elbow) for the infant to see if there is a pulse. If not, initiate CPR with chest compressions and breaths at the correct rate.

3. Adult rescue breaths are given at the rate of one per 5 seconds; children 8 and below are given one breath every 3 seconds; infants are given one breath every 3 seconds.

4. The rate of chest compressions and breaths are as follows:
   Adult: 15 compressions to 2 breaths
   Child: 5 compressions to 1 breath
   Infant: 5 compressions to 1 breath

5. The hand placement for CPR is as follows:

Adult: one hand interlocked with the other, placed two finger widths above the sternal notch
Child: heel of one hand only; same placement as adult
Infant: place index finger sideways between nipples with middle and ring finger resting beside it on sternum; lift the index finger and begin chest compressions with the middle and ring fingers

6. You perform the Heimlich maneuver on a conscious adult or child who is choking. This is done by placing your arms around the patient in a bear hug. Make a fist with one hand, thumb side toward the patient's chest. Place the other hand over the balled-up fist and perform an upward thrust below the ribs but above the navel. Continue until the object is expelled or the patient becomes unconscious.

7. Treatment for a choking infant consists of turning the infant prone with head downward and performing five back blows between the shoulder blades. Then you turn the infant face up but head still downward and give five chest compressions (the same hand placement as for infant CPR). This continues until the infant expels the object.

8. Treatment for an unconscious choking adult and child consists of straddling the

patient, performing up to five upward thrusts in the same area as the Heimlich maneuver; then performing blind finger sweeps in an adult, but in a child, inspecting the mouth for any foreign object and performing a finger sweep only if something is seen.

9. A patient could have a heart attack without realizing it. Sometimes the symptoms may be mild, and the patient may think it is only indigestion.

10. The type of burn without any blistering is a first-degree burn.

11. Measures to take when a person is bleeding are as follows:

Place direct pressure on the site of bleeding. If bleeding soaks through the pad, another pad should be applied on top of the first pad so as not to disrupt the clotting process. Elevate the area. Use pressure points. If all else fails and it becomes a matter of life or death, apply a tourniquet.

12. A victim of shock will have a very low blood pressure or unobtainable blood pressure.

13. The first step in a poisoning case is to dilute the poison by giving the patient liquids to drink.

14. A fracture with the bone piercing through the skin is a compound fracture.

15. Squeezing the stinger in an insect bite is contraindicated because the venom is then more likely to spread in that area.

16. Dry, flushed skin is indicative of a diabetic coma.

17. Syncope is another term for fainting.

NOTES:

SITE LICENSE

<u>Software Diskette to Accompany MEDICAL ASSISTANT REVIEW by Marsha Perkins Hemby</u>
PH Career & Technology

YOU SHOULD CAREFULLY READ THE FOLLOWING TERMS AND CONDITIONS BEFORE OPENING THIS DISKETTE PACKAGE. OPENING THIS DISKETTE PACKAGE INDICATES YOUR ACCEPTANCE OF THESE TERMS AND CONDITIONS. IF YOU DO NOT AGREE WITH THEM, YOU SHOULD PROMPTLY RETURN THE PACKAGE UNOPENED, AND YOUR MONEY WILL BE REFUNDED.

Prentice Hall, Inc. provides this program and licenses its use. You assume responsibility for the selection of the program to achieve your intended results, and for the installation, use, and results obtained from the program. This license extends only to use of the program in the United States or countries in which the program is marketed by duly authorized distributors.

LICENSE

You may:
a.   use the program;
b.   copy the program into any machine-readable form without limit;
c.   modify the program and/or merge it into another program in support of your use of the program.

LIMITED WARRANTY

THE PROGRAM IS PROVIDED "AS IS" WITHOUT WARRANTY OF ANY KIND, EITHER EXPRESSED OR IMPLIED, INCLUDING, BUT NOT LIMITED TO, THE IMPLIED WARRANTIES OF MERCHANTABILITY AND FITNESS FOR A PARTICULAR PURPOSE. THE ENTIRE RISK AS TO THE QUALITY AND PERFORMANCE OF THE PROGRAM IS WITH YOU. SHOULD THE PROGRAM PROVE DEFECTIVE, YOU (AND NOT PRENTICE HALL, INC. OR ANY AUTHORIZED DISTRIBUTOR) ASSUME THE ENTIRE COST OF ALL NECESSARY SERVICING, REPAIR, OR CORRECTION.

SOME STATES DO NOT ALLOW THE EXCLUSION OF IMPLIED WARRANTIES, SO THE ABOVE EXCLUSION MAY NOT APPLY TO YOU. THIS WARRANTY GIVES YOU SPECIFIC LEGAL RIGHTS AND YOU MAY ALSO HAVE OTHER RIGHTS THAT VARY FROM STATE TO STATE.

Prentice Hall, Inc. does not warrant that the function contained in the program will meet your requirements or that the operation of the program will be uninterrupted or error free.

However, Prentice Hall, Inc. warrants the diskette(s) on which the program is furnished to be free from defects in materials and workmanship under normal use for a period of ninety (90) days from the date of delivery to you as evidenced by a copy of your receipt.

LIMITATIONS OF REMEDIES

Prentice Hall's entire liability and your exclusive remedy shall be:

1.   the replacement of any diskette not meeting Prentice Hall's "Limited Warranty" and that is returned to Prentice Hall with a copy of your purchase order, or

2.   if Prentice Hall is unable to deliver a replacement diskette or cassette that is free of defects in materials or workmanship, you may terminate this Agreement by returning the program, and your money will be refunded.

IN NO EVENT WILL PRENTICE HALL BE LIABLE TO YOU FOR ANY DAMAGES, INCLUDING ANY LOST PROFITS, LOST SAVINGS, OR OTHER INCIDENTAL OR CONSEQUENTIAL DAMAGES ARISING OUT OF THE USE OR INABILITY TO USE SUCH PROGRAM EVEN IF PRENTICE HALL OR AN AUTHORIZED DISTRIBUTOR HAS BEEN ADVISED OF THE POSSIBILITY OF SUCH DAMAGES, OR FOR ANY CLAIM BY ANY OTHER PARTY.

SOME STATES DO NOT ALLOW THE LIMITATION OR EXCLUSION OF LIABILITY FOR INCIDENTAL OR CONSEQUENTIAL DAMAGES, SO THE ABOVE LIMITATION MAY NOT APPLY TO YOU.

GENERAL

You may not sublicense, assign, or transfer the license or the program except as expressly provided in this Agreement. Any attempt otherwise to sublicense, assign, or transfer any of the rights, duties, or obligations hereunder is void.

This Agreement will be governed by the laws of the State of New York.

Should you have any questions concerning this Agreement, you may contact Prentice Hall, Inc. by writing to:

Prentice Hall
Career & Technology
Englewood Cliffs, NJ 07632

YOU ACKNOWLEDGE THAT YOU HAVE READ THIS AGREEMENT, UNDERSTAND IT, AND AGREE TO BE BOUND BY ITS TERMS AND CONDITIONS. YOU FURTHER AGREE THAT IT IS THE COMPLETE AND EXCLUSIVE STATEMENT OF THE AGREEMENT BETWEEN US THAT SUPERSEDES ANY PROPOSAL OR PRIOR AGREEMENT, ORAL OR WRITTEN, AND ANY OTHER COMMUNICATIONS BETWEEN US RELATING TO THE SUBJECT MATTER OF THIS AGREEMENT.

ISBN 08359-4928-1